Overview Map Key

T0151438

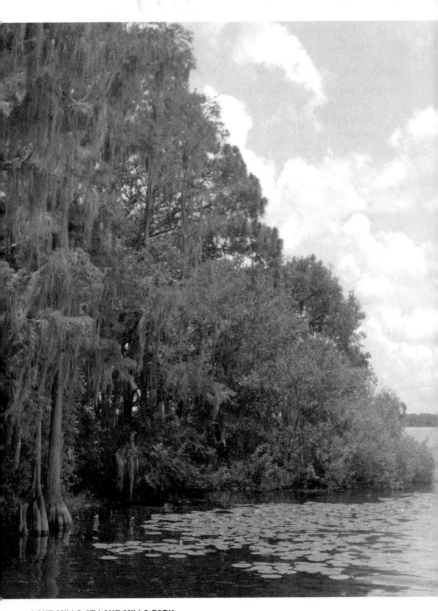

LAKE MILLS AT LAKE MILLS PARK

Five-Star Trails

Orlando

Your Guide to the Area's Most Beautiful Hikes

Sandra Friend

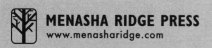
MENASHA RIDGE PRESS
www.menasharidge.com

Five-Star Trails Orlando
Your Guide to the Area's Most Beautiful Hikes

Copyright © 2012 by Sandra Friend
All rights reserved
Published by Menasha Ridge Press
Distributed by Publishers Group West
Printed in the United States of America
First edition, first printing

Cover design by Scott McGrew
Text design by Annie Long
Cover photographs by Sandra Friend
Interior photographs by Sandra Friend unless otherwise noted
Cartography by Scott McGrew
Indexing by Jan Mucciarone

ISBN: 978-0-89732-992-7

CATALOGING-IN-PUBLICATION DATA IS AVAILABLE FROM THE LIBRARY OF CONGRESS

Menasha Ridge Press
P.O. Box 43673
Birmingham, AL 35243
menasharidgepress.com

DISCLAIMER
This book is meant only as a guide to select trails in and near Orlando, Florida, and the greater metropolitan area. This book does not guarantee hiker safety in any way—you hike at your own risk. Neither Menasha Ridge Press nor Sandra Friend is liable for property loss or damage, personal injury, or death that result in any way from accessing or hiking the trails described in the following pages. Please be especially cautious when walking in potentially hazardous terrains with, for example, steep inclines or drop-offs. Do not attempt to explore terrain that may be beyond your abilities. Please read carefully the introduction to this book as well as further safety information from other sources. Familiarize yourself with current weather reports and maps of the area you plan to visit (in addition to the maps provided in this guidebook). Be cognizant of park regulations and always follow them. Do not take chances.

Contents

South   130

West   158

Northwest   182

Dedication

To John, for making me smile

Acknowledgments

Friends make hiking so much more fun, and my friends do put up with a lot—like listening to me talk into a digital recorder while I hike, stop and say *wow* a lot, and hiking at a slow enough pace that I can take data points and photos galore.

I owe a debt of gratitude to the friends who walked with me for this book. They include Joan Jarvis, Morena Cameron, G. K. Sharman, Jennifer Nelms, Ben Goldfarb, Teresa French, Tom Regan, and, especially, Paul Guyon and John Keatley for those long day hikes.

Thanks, too, to my mom, Linda Friend, and to friends from the Florida Trail Association, whose Meetups I crashed to collect trail information. A special thanks to Jim and Nancy Escoffier from the Indian River chapter and to Rodney Posey from the Central Florida chapter.

Preface

Growing up in the Appalachian Mountains, I fell in love with hiking. Life in a rural community meant a walk through the woods every day to elementary school, and it was during those meanders on my own that I'd take the time to look under rocks, smell the wildflowers, and hop from rock to rock across the creek. When my family moved to Florida in the late 1970s, we'd already spent weeks every year roaming through state parks and national parks that showcased a very different outdoors than I grew up in. But the trails in Florida led us into places that resembled the jungles I'd seen in movies. Giant spiders dangled from sticky yellow webs. Massive palm fronds slapped us in the face in the breeze. Strange rocky holes tunneled into the earth. Water bubbled up from turquoise puddles surrounded by giant trees. This was a *seriously* different place to hike.

As an adult, postcollege, my outdoor skills were honed in the Alleghenies and Appalachians, with treks along high ridges and rock scrambles. Returning to Florida in 1999, coping with the loss of my sister, I turned to the outdoors and saw it through a new set of eyes. I connected with fellow hikers in the Florida Trail Association, who taught me the fundamentals of hiking in Florida. My first lesson was "we don't hike in August." If you look at the "Weather" section (pages 8–9), you'll see why. Florida's hiking season—October through April—is flip-flopped from the rest of the country's. I hiked in August anyway. And I wrote about it. Nearly a dozen hiking guides and a busy website later, I'm still having fun sharing my Florida finds.

Orlando is the epicenter of Florida hiking, which is why I'm glad I live nearby. When the publisher asked me to put together a list of hikes for the book, they specified hikes within a two-hour driving radius from Orlando. As it turned out, I found far more than I could include within an hour's drive of downtown, thanks to the aggressive purchase of conservation lands in the past decade.

As is true through the lower peninsula of Florida, much of the Orlando region is defined by water, with rivers and streams feeding both the north-flowing St. Johns River and the south-flowing Kissimmee River. Add in the high sand ridges that were dunes along ancient shores, and the habitat diversity becomes truly spectacular. Along several hikes, you can see an unexpected marriage: tulip poplars—a well-known deciduous tree from the Appalachians, here at the southern extent of its range—with wild coffee, creeping northward from the tropics. Many of our trails, especially along the St. Johns River basin, have that jungle feel. Others lead you across wide-open prairies or tunnel into oak forests less than a dozen feet high. You'll look up at some of the most ancient cypresses in the Southeast and look down into delicate bogs brimming with carnivorous plants. You'll also have the opportunity to traverse some of the newest and

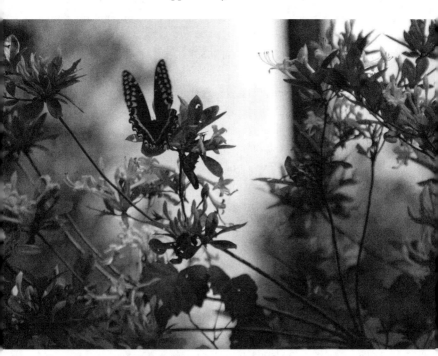

BLACK SWALLOWTAIL ON SWAMP AZALEA AT MILLS CREEK WOODLANDS

most scenic segments of the Florida Trail, our 1,400-mile National Scenic Trail, as it crosses this region.

This book is designed for hikers of all abilities. Included are some of the roughest, longest day hikes available in this mountainless region, as well as hikes of moderate length, and strolls that are perfect for families with small children or people with limited mobility. At some parks, especially in the urban areas, you can reward the kids with time on the playground after a short but beautiful walk in the woods. In the wilder places, primitive camping is available along many of the trails, enabling you to turn a day hike into a backpacking experience. All of the hikes, however, can be done in a day, with this caveat: Hikes 13 (pages 94–100), 25 (pages 165–169), and 30 (pages 195–200) are best planned with shuttle arrangements so that they don't become prohibitively long day trips; or you can follow the "Route Details" for advice on where to turn around to retrace your steps back to the starting point if you do not have a shuttle car or pickup arrangement.

Note: Always remain aware of the available, seasonal natural light for these day hikes. Be especially mindful when hiking in wooded areas, where darkness prevails earlier than on exposed trails. For example, in late November, if you are headed out on a four-hour hike described as heavily forested, do not begin the trek at 2 p.m.!

Best known as the center of Florida tourism, Orlando is a worldwide destination for families. When these visitors return for a second or third or fifteenth time, they also want to know where to play outdoors. I know, because they e-mail me all the time for suggestions. This book will outfit you for those natural getaways. In fact, while *Five-Star Trails: Orlando* focuses on hiking rather than camping, campground information is provided when a facility is available. Just look for the "Facilities" item on the opening page of each entry or the "Nearby Attractions" section at the end of each entry.

I wrote this book to connect you with nature, so you'll fall in love with our state's unique blend of ecosystems and want to protect them for future generations. Share these hikes with your family and friends to immerse them in Orlando's natural side.

Recommended Hikes

Best for Ancient Trees

7 Lake Monroe Conservation Area: Kratzert Tract (p. 60)

9 Spring Hammock Preserve (p. 70)

19 Lake Runnymede Conservation Area (p. 132)

22 Taylor Creek Loop (p. 146)

29 Blue Spring State Park: Pine Island Trail (p. 189)

Best for Birding

8 Lyonia Preserve (p. 65)

16 Orlando Wetlands Park (p. 111)

25 Lake Louisa State Park (p. 165)

Best Boardwalks

1 Black Hammock Wilderness Area (p. 26)

15 Lake Mills Park (p. 106)

26 Oakland Nature Preserve (p. 170)

33 Lake Lotus Park (p. 212)

Best for Dogs

11 Econlockhatchee Sandhills Conservation Area (p. 84)

21 Shingle Creek Regional Park: Historic Steffee Homestead (p. 141)

31 Gemini Springs Park (p. 201)

35 St. Francis Trail (p. 223)

Best for Florida Trail Segments

2 Florida Trail: Little Big Econ State Forest (p. 31)

13 Florida Trail: Bronson State Forest (p. 94)

14 Florida Trail: Mills Creek Woodlands (p. 101)

18 Tosohatchee Wildlife Management Area (p. 123)

30 Florida Trail: Seminole State Forest (p. 195)

Best for Kids

Best for Scenic Vistas

Best for Seclusion

Best for Wildflowers

Best for Wildlife

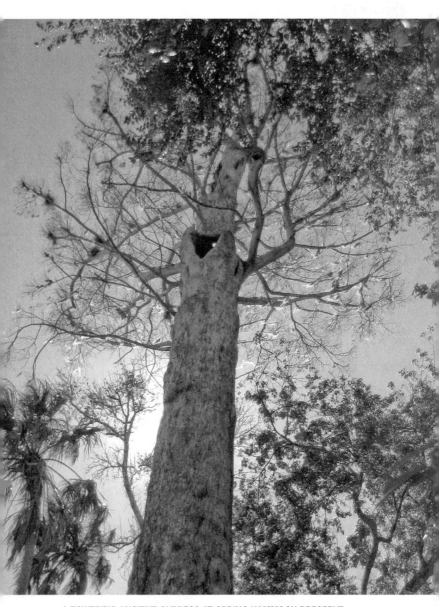

A TOWERING ANCIENT CYPRESS AT SPRING HAMMOCK PRESERVE

Introduction

About This Book

Outranked in population density only by Miami and Tampa, greater Orlando is Florida's third-largest metropolitan area. From the northern city of Sanford along the St. Johns River, to Kissimmee–St. Cloud and the Kissimmee River Basin to the south, people and development pack this region. Still, nature beckons.

Thanks to the legacy of Wiley Dykes Sr., who established a Florida Trail Association chapter in Orlando in the 1970s, local volunteers have built and maintained pathways on public lands throughout the region for more than 40 years. In more recent times, land conservation programs within the metro area have added significantly to our public lands, with volunteers and staff creating trails for public access.

To select the 37 hikes in this guide, I visited more than 50 trail systems and parks. Putting the hikes up against the *Five-Star Trails* rating system (see "Star Ratings," pages 5–6) helped me narrow them down to the best. Regarding the rating category "Scenery," panoramas in Florida are subjective: we rarely have vistas along our trails, although a few in this guidebook do offer scenics. Thus, in this category, I gave high marks to trails where you could look around and feel a part of the landscape, where the habitats immersed you in the hiking experience with few outside distractions. No hikes merit five stars in all of the rating categories, of course, because some are weighted toward, for example, wilderness experiences and others may focus on the ease of taking young children out on the trail.

These 37 hikes lie in all directions. For geographic convenience in both reading about and planning your outings, I have organized the entries in this book by their location relative to Interstate 4, which runs northeast/southwest. Hikes to the west and south lie in the theme-park areas; those in the north and east are near well-established historic communities.

Northeast of Orlando

The Econlockhatchee River reaches the St. Johns River near Lake Harney, which is part of the "River of Lakes" of the St. Johns. Proximity to these floodplain-driven waterways means spectacularly lush forests, including some with centuries-old cypress trees. Hammocks—the Florida word for patches of dense forest—are shaded by ancient live oaks and tall cabbage palms, creating a junglelike feel. Where there is elevation gain, though slight in this state, entirely different zones emerge, including pine savannas and scrub—unusual diminutive forests atop bright white sand, Florida's desert habitat. The riverfront city of Sanford, with more than 50,000 residents and a colorful historic downtown, anchors this area, acting as the interface between rural and suburban communities.

East of Orlando

Along FL 50, heading east from downtown Orlando toward Titusville, the scenery segues from strip malls to ranchland and forest as you approach Christmas. Aptly named, the community was established on Christmas Day 1837 with construction of a log fort to protect soldiers and settlers during the Second Seminole War. Thanks to the St. Johns River, natural lands surround Christmas. Florida's largest and longest river, the St. Johns cradles metro Orlando in a broad, sweeping arc to the northwest. In this area, the river's spread is wide and mazy. When it rises over its banks, it swamps across adjacent public lands, nourishing the low-lying cypress swamps, floodplain forests, and palm hammocks. The Econlockhatchee River, which flows north to the St. Johns, creates somewhat of a boundary between suburban and rural communities, where upland habitats such as pine flatwoods and sandhills are protected.

South of Orlando

Known best for its theme parks, the Kissimmee–St. Cloud area was once Florida's frontier, the jumping-off point to follow the

Kissimmee River south to Lake Okeechobee. Today, it's where urban bustle blends into cattle country, where cowboys ride across vast ranchlands, tending to herds. This section includes urban parks surrounded by suburbia, as well as an outstanding hike at Triple N Ranch (see page 151) that showcases the wide-open spaces where cattle still roam. Both Kissimmee and adjacent St. Cloud have beautiful historic downtowns with lakefront parks for urban walking.

West of Orlando

Driving west from downtown Orlando along FL 50, it's urban along the 26-mile corridor to Clermont. It takes a little searching among the suburbs to find places to hike in this least-protected part of the region. Lake Apopka, Florida's third-largest lake, sits at the base of the northernmost tip of the hilly Lake Wales Ridge. Both can be explored on the trails in this section.

Northwest of Orlando

Scarcely 6 miles northwest of downtown Orlando, feeder streams start their flow toward the Wekiva River, another major tributary of the St. Johns. Spring-fed at its source, the Wekiva is one of only two nationally designated Wild and Scenic Rivers in Florida. Suburbia, through Longwood and Apopka, runs right up to the edge of the 42,000 acres of public lands that protect the river basin. Karst features, created by the dissolution of limestone by water running over oak leaves, are common. Upland areas near Blackwater Creek include vast prairies and pine savannas, with more dense hammocks as you near the St. Johns River again. Established in 1882, DeLand, a college town with 27,000 residents, sits at the northwest corner of this section.

How To Use This Guidebook

The following information walks you through this guidebook's organization to make it easy and convenient to plan great hikes.

Overview Map, Map Key, and Map Legend

The overview map on the inside front cover depicts the location of the primary trailhead for each of the 37 hikes described in this book. The numbers shown on the overview map correspond to the map key on the facing page. Each hike's number remains with that hike throughout the book, so if you spot an appealing hiking area on the overview map, you can flip through and find those hikes easily by their sequential numbers at the top of each entry's opener page.

Trail Maps

In addition to the overview map on the inside cover, a detailed map of each hike's route appears with its profile. On each of these maps, symbols indicate the trailhead, the complete route, significant features, facilities, and topographic landmarks such as creeks, overlooks, and peaks. A legend identifying the map symbols used throughout the book appears on the inside back cover.

To produce the highly accurate maps in this book, I used a handheld GPS unit to gather data while hiking each route, and then sent that data to the publisher's expert cartographers. However, your GPS is not a substitute for sound, sensible navigation that takes into account the conditions that you observe while hiking.

Further, despite the high quality of the maps in this guidebook, the publisher and I strongly recommend that you always carry an additional map, such as the ones noted in each entry opener's listing for "Maps."

Elevation

You will note that I have not listed elevation readings in the at-a-glance information that introduces each hike, nor has the publisher included any elevation profiles. The highest point in the state of Florida is documented to be the Panhandle's Britton Hill, at 345 feet. Thus, the publisher and I agreed that including elevation in this book was not necessary to help you plan or engage in Orlando-area hiking.

The Hike Profile

Each profile opens with the hike's star ratings, GPS trailhead coordinates, and other at-a-glance information, such as the trail's distance and configuration and contacts for local information. Each profile also includes a map (see "Trail Maps," above). The main text for each profile includes four sections: "Overview," "Route Details," "Nearby Attractions," and "Directions" (for driving to the trailhead area). Below is an explanation of each of these elements.

Star Ratings

Five-Star Trails is a Menasha Ridge Press guidebook series geared to specific cities across the United States, such as this one for Orlando. Following is the explanation for the rating system of one to five stars in each of the five categories for each hike.

FOR SCENERY:

★ ★ ★ ★ ★	Unique or picturesque panoramas
★ ★ ★ ★	Diverse vistas
★ ★ ★	Pleasant views
★ ★	Unchanging landscape
★	Not selected for scenery

FOR TRAIL CONDITION:

★ ★ ★ ★ ★	Consistently well maintained
★ ★ ★ ★	Stable, with no surprises
★ ★ ★	Average terrain to negotiate
★ ★	Inconsistent, with good and poor areas
★	Rocky, overgrown, or often muddy

FOR CHILDREN:

★ ★ ★ ★ ★	Babes in strollers are welcome
★ ★ ★ ★	Fun for anyone past the toddler stage
★ ★ ★	Good for young hikers with proven stamina
★ ★	Not enjoyable for children
★	Not advisable for children

FOR DIFFICULTY:

★ ★ ★ ★ ★   Grueling

★ ★ ★ ★   Strenuous

★ ★ ★   Moderate (won't beat you up—but you'll know you've been hiking)

★ ★   Comfortable

★   Good for a relaxing stroll

FOR SOLITUDE:

★ ★ ★ ★ ★   Positively tranquil

★ ★ ★ ★   Spurts of isolation

★ ★ ★   Moderately secluded

★ ★   Crowded on weekends and holidays

★   Steady stream of individuals and/or groups

GPS Trailhead Coordinates

As noted in "Trail Maps," above, I used a handheld GPS unit to obtain geographic data and sent the information to the publisher's cartographers. In the opener for each hike profile, the coordinates—the intersection of the latitude (north) and longitude (west)—will orient you from the trailhead. In some cases, you can drive within viewing distance of a trailhead. Other hiking routes require a short walk to the trailhead from a parking area.

You will also note that this guidebook uses the degree–decimal minute format for presenting the GPS coordinates. The latitude and longitude grid system is likely quite familiar to you, but here is a refresher, pertinent to visualizing the GPS coordinates:

Imaginary lines of latitude—called parallels and approximately 69 miles apart—run horizontally around the globe. The equator is established to be 0°, and each parallel is indicated by degrees from it: up to 90°N at the North Pole, and down to 90°S at the South Pole.

Imaginary lines of longitude—called meridians—run perpendicular to latitude lines. Longitude lines are likewise indicated by degrees. Starting from 0° at the Prime Meridian in Greenwich, England, they continue to the east and west until they meet 180° later at the International Date Line in the Pacific Ocean. At the equator, longitude lines are also approximately 69 miles apart, but that distance narrows as the meridians converge toward the North and South Poles.

To convert GPS coordinates given in degrees, minutes, and seconds to the degree–decimal minute format used in this book, the seconds are divided by 60. For more on GPS technology, visit **usgs.gov.**

Distance & Configuration

Distance notes the length of the hike round-trip, from start to finish. If the hike description includes options to shorten or extend the hike, those round-trip distances will also be factored in. *Configuration* defines the trail as a loop, an out-and-back (taking you in and out via the same route), a figure eight, or a balloon.

Hiking Time

Two miles per hour is a general rule of thumb for the hiking times noted. That pace typically allows time for taking photos, dawdling and admiring views, and alternating stretches of hills and descents. When deciding whether to follow a particular trail, consider your pace, weather, general physical condition, and energy level that day, as well as the description of the terrain along the route. In areas prone to flooding, expect no better than 1 mile per hour if you are wading.

Highlights

Geologic or botanical features, historic sites, or other unique points of interest are emphasized.

Access

Fees or permits required to hike the trail, along with trail-access hours, are detailed here.

Maps

Resources for maps, in addition to those in this guidebook, are listed here. As previously noted, the publisher and I recommend that you carry more than one map—and that you consult those maps before heading out on the trail in order to resolve any confusion or discrepancy.

Facilities

This item alerts you to restrooms, picnic tables, campgrounds, playgrounds, and other amenities at or near the trailhead.

Wheelchair Access

At a glance, you'll see if there are paved sections or other areas for safely using a wheelchair.

Comments

Here you will find assorted nuggets of information, such as whether dogs are allowed on the trails.

Contacts

Listed here are phone numbers and websites for checking trail conditions and other day-to-day information.

Overview, Route Details, Nearby Attractions, and Directions

These four elements provide the main text about the hike. "Overview" gives you a quick summary of what to expect on the trail; "Route Details" guides you on the hike, start to finish; "Nearby Attractions" suggests appealing area sites, such as restaurants, museums, and other trails; and "Directions" gets you to the trailhead from a well-known road or highway.

Weather

Winter provides optimal hiking weather for Orlando, but we stretch it a bit to include fall and spring because of the magnificent wildflowers that bloom during those seasons. It's always a joy when the first frost comes along, since it means the insects won't trouble us for a couple of months. As the heat is intense and rains fall heavily during the summer months—when afternoon thundershowers are the norm—any summer hiking should start soon after daybreak and be completed before noon. Since so many of the trails in this region are in floodplains, if there has been rain recently in the metro area or points south, check ahead regarding river flooding to avoid having to wade through a trail.

The following chart lists average temperatures and precipitation by month for the Orlando area. For each month, "Hi Temp" is the average daytime high, "Lo Temp" is the average nighttime low, and "Rain" is the average precipitation.

MONTHLY WEATHER AVERAGES FOR ORLANDO, FLORIDA			
MONTH	HI TEMP	LO TEMP	RAIN
January	71°F	49°F	2.3"
February	74°F	52°F	2.5"
March	78°F	56°F	3.8"
April	83°F	60°F	2.7"
May	88°F	66°F	3.5"
June	91°F	72°F	7.6"
July	92°F	74°F	7.3"
August	92°F	74°F	7.1"
September	90°F	73°F	6.1"
October	85°F	66°F	3.3"
November	79°F	59°F	2.2"
December	73°F	52°F	2.6"

Water

How much is enough? In Florida, the humidity tricks you into thinking you don't need to drink more water, when in fact you do. A hiker walking steadily in 90°F heat needs approximately 10 quarts of fluid per day, or 2.5 gallons. I carry a minimum of a liter for every 4 miles I hike, and double that when the temperatures rise above 80°F. It's always smart to hydrate before your hike and make sure you have water (in a cooler) in your car when you return to the trailhead. For most people, the pleasures of hiking make carrying water a relatively minor price to pay to remain safe and healthy. So pack more water than you anticipate needing, even for short hikes.

If you are tempted to drink surface water, do so with extreme caution. Agricultural runoff can be an issue in this region, and swamp water teems with little creatures. Drinking such water presents risks for thirsty trekkers. Giardia parasites contaminate many water sources and cause the dreaded intestinal giardiasis that can last for weeks after ingestion. For information, visit the Centers for Disease Control website at **cdc.gov/parasites/giardia.**

Effective treatment is essential before using any water source found along the trail. Boiling water for 2–3 minutes is always a safe measure for camping, but day hikers can consider iodine tablets, approved chemical mixes, filtration units rated for giardia, and UV filtration. Some of these methods (for example, filtration with an added carbon filter) remove bad tastes typical in stagnant water, while others add their own taste. As a precaution, carry a means of water purification to help in a pinch if you realize you have underestimated your consumption needs.

Clothing

Weather, unexpected trail conditions, fatigue, extended hiking duration, and wrong turns can individually or collectively turn a great outing into a very uncomfortable one at best—and a life-threatening one at worst. Thus, proper attire plays a key role in staying comfortable and, sometimes, in staying alive. Here are some helpful guidelines.

★ Choose silk, wool, or synthetics for maximum comfort in all of your hiking attire—from hat to socks. Cotton is fine if the weather remains dry and stable, but you won't be happy if that material gets wet.

★ Always wear a hat, or at least tuck one into your day pack or hitch it to your belt. Hats offer all-weather sun and wind protection as well as warmth if it turns cold.

★ Wear running shoes, hiking boots, or sturdy hiking sandals with toe protection. Flip-flopping along a paved urban greenway is one thing, but never hike a trail in open sandals or casual sneakers. Your bones and arches need support, and your skin needs protection.

★ Pair that footwear with good socks. If you prefer not to sheathe your feet when wearing hiking sandals, tuck the socks into your day pack; you may need them if you get tired of sand between your toes.

★ Raingear is an absolute must in Florida, even if the day starts out clear and sunny. Tuck into your day pack, or tie around your waist, a jacket that is breathable and either water-resistant or waterproof.

Essential Gear

What's in your pack? The following list includes never-hike-without-them items, in alphabetical order, as all are equally important.

★ Extra food (trail mix, granola bars, or other high-energy foods)

★ First-aid kit, personalized to your needs

★ Flashlight or headlamp with extra bulb and batteries

★ Hat

★ Insect repellent, especially in summer (Spray beforehand, too!)

★ Map and compass or GPS. If you use a GPS, always remember to take a data point where your car is parked so you can find it again. Spare batteries are a must, too.

★ Raingear

★ Sunglasses

★ Sunscreen (Note the expiration date.)

★ Water (As emphasized more than once in this book, bring more than you think you will drink. Depending on your destination, you may want to bring a container and iodine or a filter for purifying water in case you run out.)

★ Whistle (This little gadget will be your best friend in an emergency.)

First-Aid Kit

In addition to the items above, those below may appear overwhelming for a day hike. But any paramedic will tell you that the products listed here—in alphabetical order, because all are important—are just the basics. The reality of hiking is that you can be out for a week of backpacking and get only a mosquito bite, or you can hike for an hour, slip, and suffer a bleeding abrasion or broken bone. Fortunately, the listed items collapse into a very small space. You can also purchase a convenient, prepackaged kit at your pharmacy or online.

★ Ace bandages or Spenco joint wraps

★ Antibiotic ointment (Neosporin or the generic equivalent)

★ Athletic tape

★ Band-Aids

★ Benadryl or the generic equivalent, diphenhydramine (in case of allergic reactions)

★ Blister kit (such as Moleskin or Spenco Second Skin)

★ Butterfly-closure bandages

★ Epinephrine in a prefilled syringe (typically by prescription only, for people known to have severe allergic reactions to insect stings)

★ Gauze (one roll and six 4-by-4-inch pads)

★ Hydrogen peroxide or iodine

★ Ibuprofen or acetaminophen

Note: Consider your intended terrain and the number of hikers in your party before you exclude any item cited above. A walk in an urban park may not inspire you to carry a complete kit, but anything beyond that warrants precaution. When hiking alone, you should always be prepared for a medical need. And if you are hiking with a friend or with a group, one or more people in your party should be equipped with first-aid supplies.

General Safety

The following tips may have the familiar ring of your mother's voice.

★ Always let someone know where you will be hiking and how long you expect to be gone. It's a good idea to give that person a copy of your route, particularly if you are headed into any isolated area. Let them know when you return.

★ Always sign in and out of any trail registers provided. Don't hesitate to comment on the trail condition if space is provided; that's your opportunity to alert others to any problems you encounter.

★ Do not count on a cell phone for your safety. Reception may be spotty or nonexistent on the trail, even on an urban walk—especially if it is embraced by towering trees.

★ Always carry food and water, even for a short hike. And bring more water than you think you will need. (That cannot be said often enough!)

★ Ask questions. State forest and park employees are there to help. It's a lot easier to solicit advice before a problem occurs, and it will help you avoid a mishap away from civilization when it's too late to amend an error.

★ Stay on designated trails. Even on the most clearly marked trails, there is usually a point where you have to stop and consider which path to take. If you become disoriented, don't panic. As soon as you think you may be off track, stop, assess your current direction, and then retrace your steps to the point where you went astray. Using a map, a compass, and this book, and keeping in mind what you have passed thus far, reorient yourself, and trust your judgment on which way to go. If you become absolutely unsure of how to continue, return to your vehicle the way you came in. Should you become completely lost and have no idea how to find the trailhead, remaining in place along the trail and waiting for help is most often the best option for adults and always the best option for children.

★ Always carry a whistle, another precaution that cannot be overemphasized. It may be a lifesaver if you do become lost or sustain an injury.

★ Be especially careful when wading into water. Whether you are fording a stream or sloshing across a flooded trail, make every step count. If you have any doubt about maintaining your balance, use a trekking pole or stout stick for balance. If the water seems too deep to wade, turn back. Whatever is on the other side is not worth risking your life.

★ Be careful along shorelines and bluffs. While these areas may provide spectacular views, they are potentially hazardous. Stay back from the edge of bluffs, and make absolutely sure of your footing; a misstep can mean a nasty and possibly fatal fall. Shorelines of rivers and marshes may have alligators and snakes sunning along them.

★ Standing dead trees and storm-damaged living trees pose a significant hazard to hikers. These trees may have loose or broken limbs that could fall at any time. While walking beneath trees, and when choosing a spot to rest or enjoy your snack, look up!

★ Know the symptoms of subnormal body temperature, or hypothermia. Shivering and forgetfulness are the two most common indicators of this stealthy killer. Yes, hypothermia can occur in Florida, even in the summer, especially when the hiker is wearing lightweight cotton clothing that gets wet. If symptoms present themselves, get to shelter, hot liquids, and dry clothes as soon as possible.

★ Know the symptoms of heat exhaustion (hyperthermia). Lightheadedness and loss of energy are the first two indicators. If you feel these symptoms, find some shade, drink your water, remove as many layers of clothing as practical, and stay put until you cool down. Marching through heat exhaustion leads to heatstroke—which can be fatal. If you should be sweating and you're not, that's the signature warning sign. Your hike is over at that point—heatstroke is a life-threatening condition that can cause seizures, convulsions, and eventually death. If you or a companion reaches that point, do whatever can be done to cool the victim down and seek medical attention immediately.

★ Most important of all, take along your brain. A cool, calculating mind is the single most important asset on the trail. It allows you to think before you act.

★ In summary: Plan ahead. Watch your step. Avoid accidents before they happen. Enjoy a rewarding and relaxing hike.

Watchwords for Flora and Fauna

Hikers should remain aware of the following concerns regarding plants and wildlife, described in alphabetical order.

Alligators

Alligators are the number-one fear for hikers new to Florida. But compared to encountering a grizzly (brown bear)—not possible in Florida anyway—I'll take an alligator stretched across a trail any day! Alligators are rarely a threat to humans, unless the reptiles have been fed by people and associate them with food. That means when you're hiking, you should never throw your food scraps into a body of water or near it. Pack out all food and scraps or get a friend to eat the leftovers. It also means being careful where you hike with a dog. If you are hiking in a swampy area, never bring along a dog—especially a small one.

Most alligators move out of your way when they hear you coming. But if an alligator is on the footpath and refuses to move after you've made a lot of noise—banging a hiking stick on the ground might help—don't walk up close to the animal. Give it a wide berth, circling *far* around its tail end so the gator doesn't feel trapped or threatened.

Biting Flies

When a deerfly or a horsefly bites, it feels like a chunk of your skin is being gouged out. Yellow flies, which lurk in deeply shaded areas, go for the head and shoulders and can drive you right off the trail. During unusually wet seasons, black flies emerge in small numbers, eager to harass. Covering your skin and using liberal amounts of insect repellent are your best means of protection. Even then, you'll still probably get bites. All of the biting flies appear during the summer months—another reason why it is best to hike at any other time of year in Florida.

Black Bears

Although no hiker has ever been attacked by a Florida black bear, the sight or approach of a bear can give anyone a start. If you encounter a bear while hiking, remain calm and avoid running in any direction. Make loud noises to scare off the bear, and back away slowly.

In primitive and remote areas, assume bears are present. They are common in Seminole State Forest, for instance, and throughout the Wekiva River basin. In more developed sites, check the current bear situation prior to hiking. Most encounters are food-related, as bears have an exceptional nose for food and not particularly discriminating palates. This is of greater concern to backpackers and campers, but on a day hike, you may plan a lunchtime picnic or munch on an energy bar from time to time. So remain aware and alert.

Mosquitoes

Mosquitoes, as you'd imagine, grow bigger here in Florida, and there are 80 different species just waiting to bug you. They're not just a summer annoyance—I've been bitten in the middle of December in a warm year. Mosquitoes are primarily found in deeply shaded areas and are worst at dawn and dusk. Ward them off with insect repellent and/or repellent-treated clothing. In some areas of Florida, mosquitoes are known to carry the West Nile virus, so take all due caution to avoid their bites.

Poison Ivy, Oak, and Sumac

Recognizing and avoiding poison ivy, oak, and sumac is the most effective way to prevent the painful, itchy rashes associated with these plants. Poison ivy occurs as a vine or ground cover, three leaflets to a leaf, and is common in hardwood hammocks and floodplain forests. Sometimes the vines, which can climb well up into the canopy on tree trunks, grow so large that the leaves can be mistaken for hickory leaves up above you. Poison oak has three leaflets. Poison sumac flourishes in swampland, each leaf having 7–13 leaflets. Urushiol, the oil in the sap of these plants, is responsible for the rash. Within 14 hours of exposure, raised lines or blisters appear on the affected area, accompanied by a terrible itch. Refrain from scratching, because bacteria under your fingernails can cause an infection. Wash and dry the affected area thoroughly and apply a calamine lotion to help dry

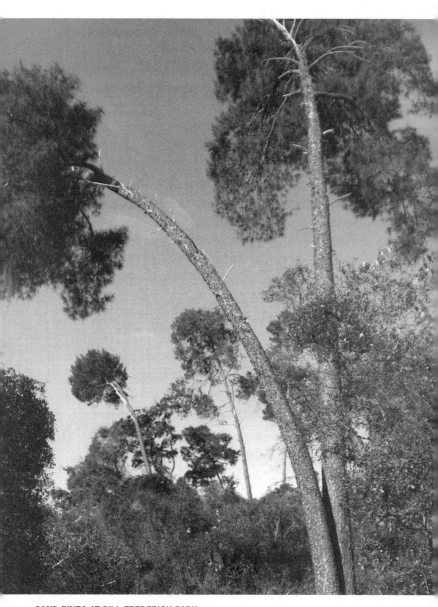

SAND PINES AT BILL FREDERICK PARK

out the rash. If itching or blistering is severe, seek medical attention. If you do come into contact with one of these plants, remember that oil-contaminated clothes, hiking gear, and pets can easily transfer the irritant to you or someone else, so wash not only any exposed parts of your body but also any exposed clothes, gear, and pets.

Snakes

Florida has six species of venomous snakes, and you could spot five of them in the Orlando region. Those five are the pygmy rattlesnake, eastern diamondback rattlesnake, timber rattlesnake, cottonmouth, and coral snake. Rattlesnakes like to bask in the sun and won't bite unless threatened. Cottonmouths are extremely territorial and will hold their ground.

The snakes you are most likely to see while hiking are non-venomous species and subspecies, with black snakes and rat snakes being the most common. The best rule is to leave all snakes alone, give them a wide berth as you hike past, and make sure any hiking companions (including dogs) do the same.

When hiking, stick to well-used trails and wear over-the-ankle boots and loose-fitting long pants. Do not step or put your hands beyond your range of detailed visibility, and avoid wandering around in the dark. Step *onto* logs and rocks, never *over* them, and be especially careful when climbing rocks. Always avoid walking through dense brush or saw palmetto thickets.

Ticks

Ticks are often found on brush and tall grass, where they seem to be waiting to hitch a ride on a warm-blooded passerby. Adult ticks are most active October through May, paralleling Florida's hiking season. Among the varieties of ticks, the black-legged tick, commonly called the deer tick, is the primary carrier of Lyme disease. Wear light-colored clothing, making it easier for you to spot ticks before they migrate to your skin. At the end of the hike, visually check your hair, the back of your neck, your armpits, and your socks. During your post-hike shower, take a moment to do a more complete body check. For ticks that are already embedded, removal with tweezers is best. Use disinfectant solution on the wound.

Hunting

Separate rules, regulations, and licenses govern the various types of hunting and their seasons. Though there are generally no problems, hikers may wish to forgo their trip during general gun season (deer season) in late fall and early winter, when the woods suddenly seem filled with orange and camouflage. For specific hunting-season dates on public lands, visit the Florida Fish and Wildlife Conservation Commission website at **myfwc.com.**

Regulations

Regulations vary among land management agencies throughout the region, with additional regulations piled onto some lands that are jointly managed by county and water management districts. Always check the trail kiosk when you arrive at a trailhead. The following agencies adhere to certain regulations year-round.

Florida State Forests

★ Primitive camping requires a permit in advance and a fee.

★ Hunting or fishing requires a valid Florida fishing license, available from the Florida Fish and Wildlife Conservation Commission.

Florida State Parks

★ Day-use hours are 8 a.m.–sunset.

★ Pets must be leashed.

★ Hunting is prohibited.

★ Fishing requires a valid Florida fishing license, available from the Florida Fish and Wildlife Conservation Commission.

★ Fishing, boating, swimming, and fires are allowed in designated areas only.

★ Alcoholic beverage consumption is allowed in designated areas only.

★ All plants, animals, and park property are protected. The collection, destruction, or disturbance of plants, animals, or park property is prohibited.

Orange County Environmental Protection Division, Green PLACE Program

★ Security is not provided. Use facilities at your own risk.

★ Open sunrise–sunset.

★ Access is allowed only from designated points.

★ Motor vehicles and pets are prohibited, and bicycles are prohibited at some locations.

★ Firearms and hunting are prohibited.

★ All vegetation, animals, facilities, and cultural resources are protected. It is unlawful to remove, destroy, deface, mutilate, or harass any of these resources.

★ Please dispose of all trash appropriately.

Seminole County Natural Lands

★ Access is allowed only from county-designated points at permitted times.

★ Open sunrise–sunset.

★ Motor vehicles are prohibited.

★ All plants and animals are protected. It is unlawful to remove or destroy plants or to remove, destroy, or harass animals.

★ Pets must be leashed.

★ Prohibited activities include hunting, possession of firearms, operation of motor vehicles, alcohol, camping (except in designated areas), swimming, dumping, destruction of property, posting of handbills, fires (except campfires in designated camping areas), public disturbance, sales or concessions, and construction.

Volusia County Natural Lands

★ Open sunrise–sunset.

★ Security is not provided. Use properties and facilities at your own risk.

★ Access is allowed only at designated points.

★ Motor vehicles are prohibited.

★ Pets must be leashed.

★ Possession and use of firearms or similar equipment is prohibited.

★ All trash must be disposed of in provided containers.

★ Vegetation, animals, cultural resources, and facilities are protected. It is unlawful to remove, destroy, deface, mutilate, or harass any of these resources.

★ Igniting or maintaining a fire is prohibited, except fires within provided grills.

★ Fireworks are prohibited.

★ Group camping requires a permit in advance.

Trail Etiquette

Always treat the trail, wildlife, and fellow hikers with respect. Here are some reminders.

★ Plan ahead to be self-sufficient at all times. For example, carry necessary supplies for changes in weather or other conditions. A well-planned trip brings satisfaction to you and to others.

★ Hike on open trails only.

★ In seasons or construction areas where road or trail closures are a possibility, use the websites or phone numbers shown in the "Contacts" line on the opening page for each hike to check conditions prior to heading out. Do not attempt to circumvent such closures.

★ Avoid trespassing on private land and obtain all required permits and authorizations. Leave gates as you found them or as directed by signage.

★ Be courteous to other hikers, bikers, equestrians, and others you encounter on the trails.

★ Never spook wild animals or pets. An unannounced approach, a sudden movement, or a loud noise startles most critters, and a surprised animal can be dangerous to you, to others, and to itself. Give animals plenty of space.

★ Observe the yield signs around the region's trailheads and backcountry. Typically they advise hikers to yield to horses, and bikers to yield to both horses and hikers. When encountering mounted riders on shared trails, hikers can courteously step off the trail. So the horse can see and hear you, calmly greet the riders before they reach you, and do not dart behind trees. Also resist the urge to pet horses unless you are invited to do so.

★ Stay on the existing trail and do not blaze any new trails.

★ Be sure to pack out what you pack in, leaving only your footprints. No one likes to see the trash someone else has left behind.

Tips on Hiking around Orlando

For a pleasant outdoor experience, plan to hike between October and April. Take along a field guide to help you learn about the plants and animals you encounter along the trail. A good general guide is *National Audubon Society Field Guide to Florida.*

My website, Florida Hikes, contains detailed information on plant communities seen along Florida's trails, as well as specific identifications of some of the common wildflowers, trees, and birds mentioned in this book. You'll also find photo galleries so you can sample the trails before you hike: **floridahikes.com.**

Try to avoid traveling on major highways during weekday rush hours. Traffic is especially heavy on I-4 in the mornings and evenings. South of downtown, there is a second rush hour, as the theme parks open and close about an hour or two later. Many of the hikes in this book are along scenic back roads, and I encourage you to use those back roads to traverse the region in a more relaxed manner than is typically possible on the main arteries.

The St. Johns River floods whenever it rains heavily to the south and east. Before you head out for any of the hikes within the river basin, check for notices on river levels on the St. Johns River Water Management District website: **sjrwmd.com.**

This book includes the most scenic segments of the statewide Florida Trail, a 1,400-mile National Scenic Trail (NST). It's one of only three in America that traverse a single state; the Ice Age NST in Wisconsin and the Arizona NST are the other two. While a handful of people thru-hike the trail each year, many more enjoy it on day hikes and backpacking trips along sections strung across the state from Big Cypress National Preserve near Naples to Gulf Islands National Seashore in Pensacola. The statewide Florida Trail Association brings together volunteers to build and maintain trail sections: **floridatrail.org.**

On weekends, urban parks and local state parks get very busy. Some parks, such as Kelly Park, Wekiwa Springs State Park, and Blue Spring State Park, close their gates when their parking areas reach capacity. This can happen early on Saturday mornings. If you have your heart set on doing a certain hike on a certain Saturday, get there early!

While most of the hikes in the book have no entrance fee, those in Florida State Parks do (fees are noted on each entry's "Access" line). If you're a frequent parks traveler, consider purchasing an annual pass good throughout the entire Florida State Parks system, now numbering more than 160 parks: **floridastateparks.org/thingstoknow /annualpass.cfm.**

Guided hikes are offered frequently throughout the region by volunteers with the Central Florida chapter of the Florida Trail Association. Going with a group is a great way to meet fellow hikers and learn more about other outdoor activities in the area. See Appendix C (page 242) for details.

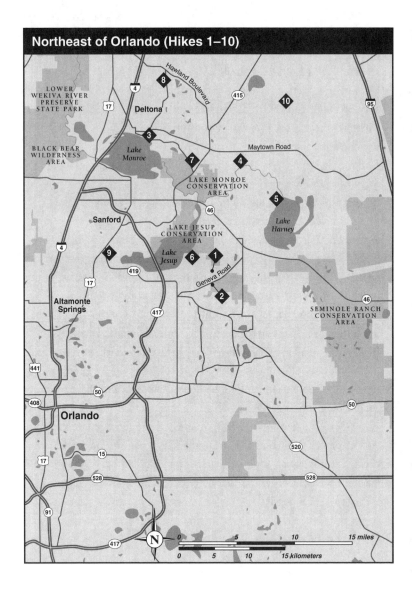

Northeast of Orlando (Hikes 1–10)

LOWER WEKIVA RIVER PRESERVE STATE PARK

Howland Boulevard

Deltona

BLACK BEAR WILDERNESS AREA

Lake Monroe

Maytown Road

LAKE MONROE CONSERVATION AREA

Sanford

LAKE JESUP CONSERVATION AREA

Lake Jesup

Lake Harney

Geneva Road

Altamonte Springs

SEMINOLE RANCH CONSERVATION AREA

Orlando

N

0   5   10   15 miles

0   5   10   15 kilometers

Northeast

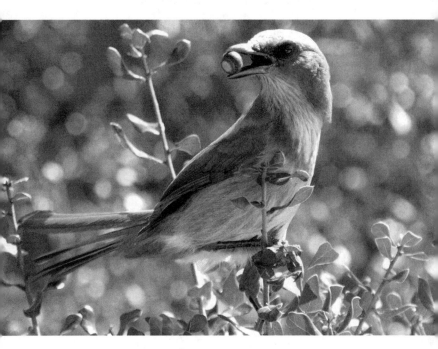

FLORIDA SCRUB-JAY AT LYONIA PRESERVE

Black Hammock Wilderness Area

SCENERY: ★ ★ ★ ★ ★
TRAIL CONDITION: ★ ★ ★
CHILDREN: ★ ★
DIFFICULTY: ★ ★ ★
SOLITUDE: ★ ★ ★

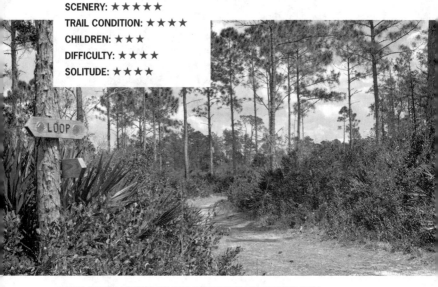

START OF THE LOOP AT BLACK HAMMOCK WILDERNESS AREA

GPS TRAILHEAD COORDINATES: N28° 41.962' W81° 09.553'

DISTANCE & CONFIGURATION: 4.5-mile balloon

HIKING TIME: 2.5 hours

HIGHLIGHTS: Long boardwalks; diverse flora habitat, including semitropical hammock; sheltered benches

ACCESS: Free; open daily, sunrise–sunset

MAPS: USGS *Oviedo*

FACILITIES: None

WHEELCHAIR ACCESS: Graded shell rock leads to a long, accessible boardwalk

COMMENTS: Limited parking; strenuous hiking in scrub portion of the trail

CONTACTS: Seminole County Natural Lands Program (407) 665-2001; **seminolecountyfl .gov/parksrec/naturallands/blackhammock.aspx**

Overview

In more than 700 acres along the rim of Lake Jesup, the trails of Black Hammock Wilderness Area provide an exploration of habitats affected by the proximity of this 25-square-mile shallow lake. Two lengthy and narrow boardwalks over a floodplain forest form a bridge to an upland hammock, pond pine flatwoods, and a loop within open scrub. While you never see the lake, which is an arm of the "River of Lakes" of the St. Johns River, its effect on the landscape is notable in the diversity of plant life along the trail.

Route Details

Leaving the parking area, stop and sign in at the kiosk, where you can pick up trail info and maps. The trail enters a diminutive scrub forest where a footpath of bright white sand and crunchy shell rock meanders among saw palmetto trees. Just beyond them are tall loblolly bay trees, providing an interesting interface of dry and wet habitats. Approaching the boardwalk, you duck under the oaks. Here, just north of Oviedo—named Tree City U.S.A. year after year and where vegetable farming has gone on for more than a century—you will see a plaque dedicating the boardwalk to Jim Logue. He was a local resident who worked to ensure the Black Hammock would remain a protected rural area as suburban sprawl crept close.

The boardwalk is such a major feature of the hike that it's worth coming out just to walk that. Narrow and long, it tunnels through the woods, carrying you a few feet above the floodplain forest. Insistent thistle rises from the forest floor to show off puffy purple blooms, and tall, spindly cabbage palms tower overhead. Your perspective is turned skyward to marvel at the canopy of trees, but take the time to peer over the railing too, to see the thickets of ferns. The boardwalk ends on an island in the floodplain, where needle palms form a backdrop beneath oaks and cabbage palms, and colorful fungi peep out from fallen logs.

As you reach a second boardwalk, look up and notice the bromeliads making the limbs of the oak trees look fuzzy. Tall cedars and

Black Hammock Wilderness Area

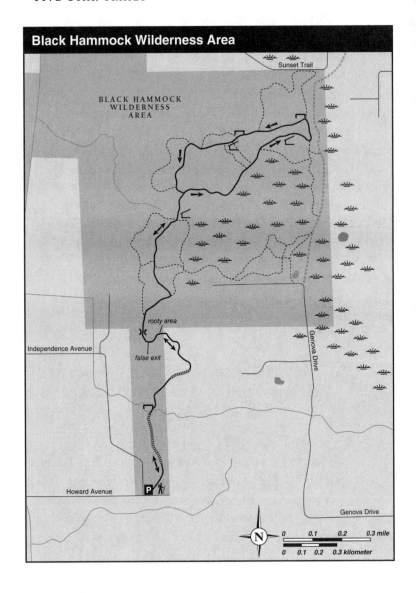

BLACK HAMMOCK
WILDERNESS
AREA

Sunset Trail

rooty area

Independence Avenue

false exit

Howard Avenue

Genova Drive

Genova Drive

N

| 0 | 0.1 | 0.2 | 0.3 mile |

| 0 | 0.1 | 0.2 | 0.3 kilometer |

loblolly pines intersperse with cabbage palms and sweetgum trees. This boardwalk drops you into a forest dense with southern magnolias. Thick bromeliads filling the upper branches of the oaks look like rows of hanging flags. By now you've discovered the natural beauty of Black Hammock, lush vegetation brought about by high humidity in the hardwood forest. Blue and silver markers indicate the distinct path.

Crossing a bridge over a creek that drains toward Lake Jesup, you've walked nearly a mile. This is where the trail begins to rise up into scrubby pine flatwoods, where there is little shade but still many songbirds. At the T-intersection, turn right. Pond pine grows along the edges of the road, distinctive with its needles seeming to pop out of the tree trunks. At the fork, turn left, following the arrow. The sand gets soft underfoot. If you are here in springtime, you will note the gallberry shrubs sporting their magenta blooms.

At 1.4 miles you reach a trail junction. Continue straight to a large bridge over an ephemeral waterway and a bench soon after. Immediately after the bench, there's a trail junction. Keep right to find the well-marked start of a 1.7-mile path that loops through pine flatwoods and scrub, back to this junction. (As you follow the trail, watch for the trail markers, as the scrub forest is crisscrossed with firebreaks and alternative trails where you can get pretty lost if you don't carefully stay to the main route.) The trail goes through an area that gets seasonally wet, so dress accordingly. A little elevation gain and you're into the scrub, with Chapman and myrtle oak growing in the white sand and no shade overhead.

At 2.1 miles, after you pass a prairie on the left, you will spot a bench for a quick rest if you want to pause. Otherwise, turn right and continue into the sand pine scrub. It looks like good Florida scrub-jay habitat, with lots of rusty lyonia. At the T-intersection, turn left. The footpath turns to soft white sand—pretty but difficult to walk in. At the next bench, the trail turns left to start back along the loop. Going left again at the next fork, the trail drops back into pond pine flatwoods, thankfully out of the sugar-soft sand. Go straight ahead at the next trail junction.

Coming around a corner framed by young pond pines, you reach another bench at 2.6 miles. Pines close in more thickly, and the walls of saw palmetto rise taller as the trail continues its moderate descent. At the unmarked fork in the trail, turn left and look for an arrow on a pine tree, a confirmation blaze. At the next intersection, you've completed the loop. Turn right and you'll see the back side of the sign marking the beginning of the loop.

At 3.1 miles pass the bridge to start your return to the boardwalk. Watch for the trail markers to guide you back through the scrubby flatwoods. When you see a house to the right, keep left at that fork to head back into the delightful shade of the hardwood hammock, following the trail as it winds back around the small bridge. Around 3.6 miles it appears that the trail goes straight into the woods at a place where there is some graffiti on a tree. Turn left to stay on the main trail. Once you're back on the boardwalk, your route is obvious. Savor the views on your way back to the trailhead.

Nearby Attractions

Lake Jesup Conservation Area (Hike 6, page 54) is within close proximity to this hike and provides a place to see the lake, as does the funky fish camp, Black Hammock Adventures, at the other point of this dead-end road. Along with fishing, this lively nightspot includes live alligators, airboat rides, a tiki bar on Lake Jesup, and an excellent seafood restaurant. Visit **theblackhammock.com.**

Directions

From FL 417, Exit 44, follow FL 434 toward Oviedo. After 1 mile, turn left at the Black Hammock sign on the curve onto DeLeon Street. Continue down DeLeon Street to a T at Howard Avenue. Turn right onto Howard Avenue and drive 3 miles to its end, where the road narrows. Please drive slowly, as there may be equestrians or children on the road. Be respectful of private property along the road and park only in the parking corral at the trailhead.

2 Florida Trail: Little Big Econ State Forest

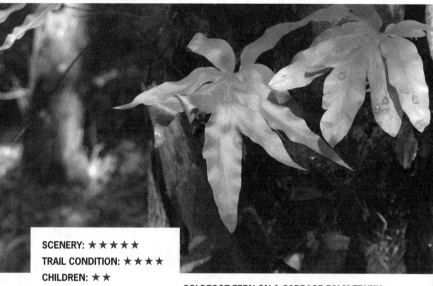

SCENERY: ★ ★ ★ ★ ★
TRAIL CONDITION: ★ ★ ★ ★
CHILDREN: ★ ★
DIFFICULTY: ★ ★ ★ ★
SOLITUDE: ★ ★ ★ ★

GOLDFOOT FERN ON A CABBAGE PALM TRUNK

GPS TRAILHEAD COORDINATES: N28° 41.242' W81° 09.553'

DISTANCE & CONFIGURATION: 4.5-mile out-and-back

HIKING TIME: 3.5 hours

HIGHLIGHTS: River bluffs, scenic views, crossed palms

ACCESS: $2 per person day-use fee; open 24/7

MAPS: USGS *Oviedo* and *Geneva*

FACILITIES: None

WHEELCHAIR ACCESS: None

COMMENTS: Leashed pets are allowed, and camping is by permit only. Do not hike this trail when the river is in flood stage.

CONTACTS: Little Big Econ State Forest (407) 971-3500; **floridaforestservice.com/state_forests/little_big_econ.html**

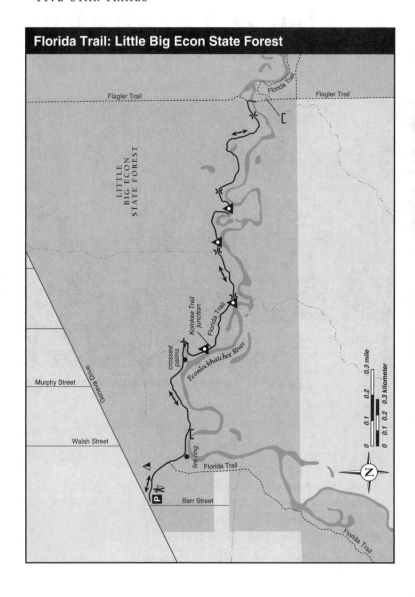

Florida Trail: Little Big Econ State Forest

Flagler Trail

Flagler Trail

Florida Trail

LITTLE
BIG ECON
STATE FOREST

Kolokee Trail junction

Florida Trail

crossed palms

Econlockhatchee River

Geneva Drive

Murphy Street

Walsh Street

fire ring

Florida Trail

Barr Street

Florida Trail

0.3 mile

0.3 kilometer

0.1   0.2

0   0.1   0.2

0

N

Overview

Amid the Little Big Econ State Forest, a ribbon of wilderness holds the line between rural life and suburbia northeast of Orlando. Here, the statewide Florida Trail shows off along a particularly beautiful segment of the Econlockhatchee (Econ) River. Following the river bluffs several miles east from the Barr Street Trailhead in Oviedo, this piece of trail is well loved by day hikers and backpackers alike. Rugged yet easy to follow, it's a satisfying walk in the woods to a river crossing that connects with the multiuse Flagler Trail.

Route Details

Starting from the trailhead kiosk, a white-blazed approach trail connects to the Florida Trail. It enters a leafy hardwood hammock, where a side trail leads to a tent-camping area in an open meadow. Losing a little elevation, the trail drops down through scrub habitat to the T-intersection with the orange-blazed Florida Trail. Turn left to cross a footbridge over Salt Creek. The trail emerges into a former pasture planted in pines. It makes a right turn to stay close to the creek basin, overlooking the Econlockhatchee River at a fire ring and bench on a bluff. The river is tannic but clear, flowing in a deep channel between its high, sandy banks. Because it captures the flow of many feeder streams, it rises quickly after a heavy rain.

Turn left at the campsite. Shaded by overhanging trees, the trail follows the river bluffs. At 0.4 mile, a bench overlooks a bend of the river where Virginia willows crowd the far shore. Keep alert for the orange blazes so you don't stray off the path.

You reach a fork where it seems you should follow the river, but the Florida Trail turns left, and for good reason, as a tributary flows down to the river straight ahead. Making its way around the tributary, the trail rejoins the old pasture. You pass the first of many markers with a code number indicating your location. In case of emergency, hikers can dial 911 to summon assistance to any marker's specific location on the trail. Although you're in a wild area, the markers are a reminder that the urban mass is just a few miles away. Beyond the next primitive campsite, the trail curves to the right.

What lies before you is a diverse blend of attractions. Gleaming brilliant green in the morning light after a refreshing nighttime rain, resurrection fern covers the outstretched arms of live oaks. If there has been no rain, you will spot the dry ferns curled up on themselves. Side trails lead to river views, and you may make brief forays if you wish. But return to the main trail, which plays tag with the forest road briefly before it heads into the shady river-bluff forest. Look down to the right and you'll see a landmark along this trail, the crossed palms. Three cabbage palms are interlaced across the waterway, as if planted to grow together that way. The trail continues up this tributary, which you will cross when you reach a bridge. While the creek beneath is shallow, like the river it lies deep below, inside its sandy floodplain channel.

Pushing palm fronds aside as if you're walking through a jungle, you come to a point where the trail curves to the right and follows the creek along a narrow path between the tall palms. The star-shaped leaves of sweetgum intersperse with hickory trees and oaks. Sparkleberry and highbush blueberry arch over the trail as it rises into a stretch of scrub forest. The oaks are laden with bromeliads and ferns, with occasional clusters of greenfly orchids in the crooks of the oak limbs. Just after a side trail to a river overlook at 0.9 mile, you reach the junction with the **Kolokee Trail,** a white-blazed loop that is part of the Florida State Forest Trailwalker program. It leads through habitats similar to this but without the great river views. Stay with the orange blazes.

Pulling away from the river again, the trail loops around a swale filled with saw palmetto. Given its proximity to civilization, it's surprising that the forest peacefulness is laced primarily with the sounds of songbirds, crickets, and frogs.

Roots form stairs in the trail as it gets close to the next tributary. You pass an enormous slash pine with a large catface scar from turpentine tapping. Southern magnolia forms the lower canopy, fragrant in June with its dinner plate–sized blossoms. The trail works its way back to the bluffs, providing excellent views before it turns left.

You cross a bridge at 1.2 miles. As the trail returns to the bluffs, be cautious of your footing, as the path is narrow and rooty. Scrambling up roots, the trail works its way to a long footbridge across a deep channel covered in water spangles. At the far end of the bridge you will see marker LE 42, one of the locators mentioned earlier.

Emerging at another excellent view of the river, the trail turns left to follow the bluffs. Skirting a side channel with stagnated water and, typically, a cloud of mosquitoes, you climb into a small stretch of scrub habitat. Where the trail faces the river again, the view is simply beautiful. The next bridge over a tributary is another long span, with marker LE 41 on the far side. Returning to the river, the trail moves away from the bluffs edge and passes an enormous slash pine. The slippery leaves of southern magnolia carpet the footpath. Past the next marker, the trail dips down through a dry side channel. Following the next floodplain channel, the footpath snakes through the river-bluff forest as it comes up to the next bridge, which has an approach boardwalk. A cabbage palm curves out over the water in a U shape.

As you step out to the river bluff again, look up. It's one of the few spots from which you can see the big bridge over the Econ. More than a decade ago, crossing the river here meant a balancing act on swaying pieces of timber suspended by cables from old railroad trestle piers. But development of multiuse trails through the forest meant the bridge needed to serve all users, not just hikers. So this high, broad bridge over the river now enables equestrians, cyclists, hikers, and patrol rangers to connect to any of the trails.

At 2.3 miles, the north side of the bridge is the junction for many adventures. The multiuse Flagler Trail goes northeast from the bridge to end at Lake Harney Wilderness Area (Hike 5, page 48). The Florida Trail continues east along the river through the Little Big Econ State Forest, connecting with the Mills Creek Woodlands section (Hike 14, page 101), about 6 miles east. Crossing the bridge, you can follow the Flagler Trail 3 miles south down a shady straightaway to the Snow Hill Road Trailhead.

For now, cross the bridge and enjoy the view. On both sides of the river, you can see a part of the old railroad trestle, a circa 1911 spur line to Chuluota from Henry Flagler's Florida East Coast Railroad. Meant to open up this corridor to development, it was an early failed attempt at selling Florida swampland. Make your turnaround point the two benches (marked 14A and 14B) on the peninsula on the south side of the bridge and walk back north across the bridge.

On the north side of the bridge, ignore the sign that says the trailhead is 1.75 miles away, as that mileage comes up short. Turn west and start retracing your steps back along the river, heading upstream by following the orange blazes along the river bluffs. Follow the winding path back and forth from the bluffs to the bridges over the tributaries on the return trip. When you reach the fire ring atop the river bluffs, you've walked 4.2 miles. Turn right and follow the blazes along the edge of Salt Creek back to where the Florida Trail turns away from the old pasture planted in pines and into the forest on the left, crossing one last bridge. Turn right to follow the white-blazed trail out to the parking area, completing a 4.5-mile round-trip.

Nearby Attractions

Canoe or kayak this beautiful section of the Econlockhatchee River using a public launch along Chuluota Road (County Road 419) and a takeout at Snow Hill Road. Download a map of the river from the Office of Greenways and Trails at **dep.state.fl.us/gwt/guide /designated_paddle/Econlock_guide.pdf.**

Directions

From FL 417, Exit 44, follow FL 434 toward Oviedo. After 1 mile, turn left at the Black Hammock sign on the curve onto DeLeon Street. Continue down DeLeon Street to Florida Avenue, the first turn on the right. Turn right and drive down this rural, canopied road for 2.5 miles. It makes a hard right onto Van Arsdale Street before ending at CR 426 (Geneva Road). Turn left. After 0.7 mile, the Barr Street Trailhead is on your right.

You can also access the trailhead from the intersection of FL 46 and CR 426 in Geneva, east of Sanford. Drive west on CR 426 for 4.5 miles to the Barr Street Trailhead on the left, just after a small bridge over Salt Creek.

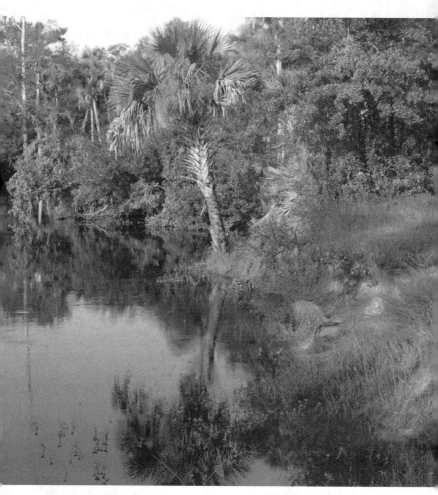

ECONLOCKHATCHEE RIVER

3 # Green Spring Park

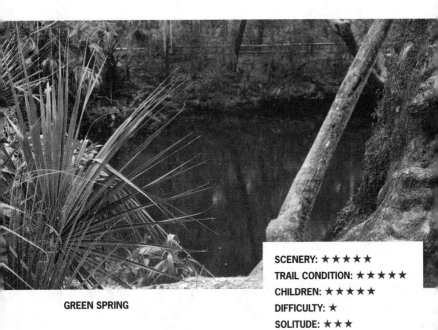

SCENERY: ★ ★ ★ ★ ★
TRAIL CONDITION: ★ ★ ★ ★ ★
CHILDREN: ★ ★ ★ ★ ★
DIFFICULTY: ★
SOLITUDE: ★ ★ ★

GREEN SPRING

GPS TRAILHEAD COORDINATES: N28° 51.789' W81° 14.912'

DISTANCE & CONFIGURATION: 0.5-mile loop and spur

HIKING TIME: 20 minutes

HIGHLIGHTS: Green Spring, ancient trees

ACCESS: Free; open daily, sunrise–sunset

MAPS: USGS *Osteen*

FACILITIES: Playground, restrooms, picnic tables and grills, paved bicycle trail

WHEELCHAIR ACCESS: Yes, using the paved trails

COMMENTS: Because of the dense shade and waterways, mosquito repellent is a must. The park is a trailhead for the Spring-to-Spring Trail, a bicycle path that connects to Gemini Springs Park (Hike 31, page 201). Leashed pets are permitted.

CONTACTS: Volusia County Government Parks, Recreation and Culture (386) 736-5953; **volusia.org/parks/green.htm**

Overview

Hidden deep in a leafy glade, a shimmering pool rises from the earth to pour through palm hammocks. At Green Spring Park, the trails are short but well groomed, with options for all abilities: both a sidewalk and a paved biking trail loop through the park, along with a network of natural footpaths. Families with small children will appreciate the tucked-in-the-woods playground and the gentle paths that sneak through the forest with surprises around each corner. Detailed, colorful interpretive signs walk you through the story of the rise and fall of Enterprise as a steamboat port on the St. Johns River.

Route Details

At the far north side of the parking area, an overview map depicts the paved concrete sidewalk around the park, as well as an asphalt bike trail. Follow the sidewalk into the woods to come across the first snippet of history about this site, the heart of the town that became Enterprise. The walkway splits around a small playground. Keep to the right, where a sign points you toward the spring. Head in that direction, crossing the bike trail, and turn right to emerge at the spring overlook.

The main spring, Green Spring, is a pretty pool set under a canopy of mature live oaks. It's not fit for swimming, nor is it clear, but it shimmers enticingly nonetheless. Its outflow goes off to your left, where an old set of stairs leads down to the spring run. A picnic table on the observation deck makes this a nice spot for a picnic lunch. To continue along the outer loop, head back the way you came, crossing the bike path to end up at the playground. Turn right.

You're walking through a palm hammock close to Lake Monroe, one of the larger lakes in the chain of lakes that makes up the St. Johns River. As the sidewalk winds through the woods, it reaches a short natural-surface path that leads along the waterway that sluices out of Green Spring. Large southern magnolias shade the channel, and sweetgum trees tower overhead. When you return to the sidewalk, turn left and make an immediate right.

Green Spring Park

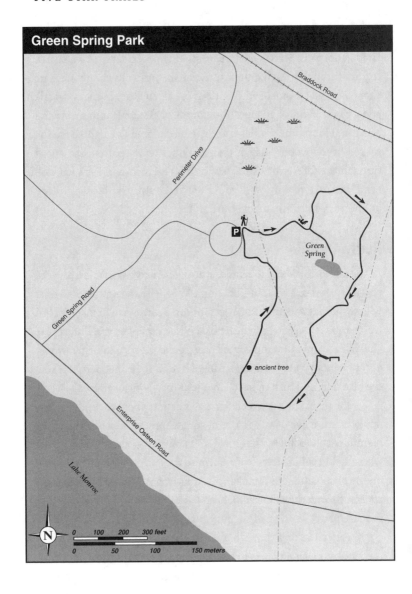

Leaving the main trail right before the bridge, continue down a short spur trail to a beauty spot where waters merge. Coming from several directions, these spring-fed trickles form a clear, winding channel. Return to the main trail and turn left. Ferns line the footpath, which is heavily shaded by the canopy of ancient trees. Another natural-surface trail comes in from the right just before this trail crosses a small bridge. Oranges dangle well out of reach overhead. As you walk down a corridor of sword ferns, the trail comes to a four-way junction. The path to the right leads back to the observation deck at the spring. Take a left. This short spur leads down to another pretty spot on the winding waterway through the palm hammock, with a bench that provides a place to sit and listen to the burble.

Return along the spur trail to the four-way intersection, and take a left. Follow the fern-lined path beneath a grapevine the width of a small tree trunk. Beautyberry sports bright purple berries in fall. Palm fronds fill the understory, as does the warble of songbirds. Passing several large cedar trees, the trail gains a little elevation, climbing into stands of hickory and elm. The footpath is strewn with fossilized snail shells, remnants of the indigenous Timucua people's midden, an ancient trash heap of tiny shells. Like most middens discovered along this river, much of it was hauled away nearly a century ago for road fill.

At 0.4 mile, the trail comes to the base of an enormous longleaf pine tree, its crown high above the rest of the forest canopy. At the T-intersection, turn left to continue on the outer loop. The canopy parts a little to reveal blue skies, but there are still many large oaks here, covered in resurrection fern and hollowed out from age. Shoelace fern dangles from the trunk of a cabbage palm.

Emerging from the junglelike palm hammock, you reach the bicycle path. Cross it and continue straight ahead onto the sidewalk, which passes between the restrooms (to your left) and a picnic shelter on the right. Continue straight ahead to the parking area to finish up the short loop.

Nearby Attractions

The town of Enterprise offers interesting architecture and a rich history; visit **oldenterprise.org.** A little farther north along Lakeshore Drive is Mariner's Cove Park, with access to Lake Monroe for boating and paddling; visit **volusia.org/parks/mariner.htm.**

Directions

From I-4, Exit 108, drive east on DeBary Avenue for 0.5 mile, where it turns into Jacob Brock Avenue for the next 0.7 mile. Turn right onto Main Street and continue through the historic town of Enterprise. Main Street jogs south to become Lakeshore Drive, which parallels the shoreline of Lake Monroe. Continue 1.1 miles to the park entrance on the left, Green Springs Road. Drive in the main gate and park along the circle.

Hickory Bluff Preserve

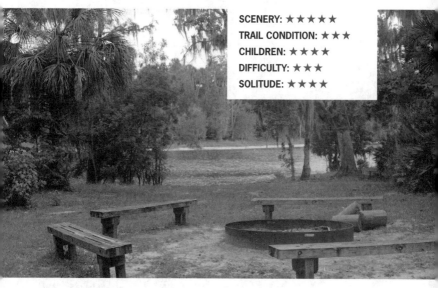

SCENERY: ★ ★ ★ ★ ★
TRAIL CONDITION: ★ ★ ★
CHILDREN: ★ ★ ★ ★
DIFFICULTY: ★ ★ ★
SOLITUDE: ★ ★ ★ ★

CAMPSITE AT HICKORY BLUFF PRESERVE

GPS TRAILHEAD COORDINATES: N28° 49.933' W81° 07.116'

DISTANCE & CONFIGURATION: 1.5-mile loop

HIKING TIME: 45 minutes

HIGHLIGHTS: Views of the St. Johns River

ACCESS: Free; open daily, sunrise–sunset

MAPS: USGS *Osceola*

FACILITIES: Group campsite, portable toilet, picnic pavilion with grill

WHEELCHAIR ACCESS: None

COMMENTS: Trails are shared with off-road cyclists and equestrians. Leashed pets are permitted, and group camping is available by permit.

CONTACTS: Volusia County Government Land Acquisition and Management (386) 424-6834; **volusia.org/growth/hickory.htm**

Hickory Bluff Preserve

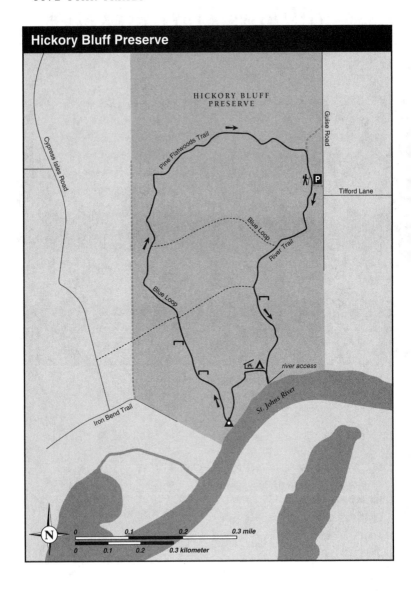

HICKORY BLUFF
PRESERVE

Pine Flatwoods Trail

Cypress Isles Road

Guise Road

Tifford Lane

Blue Loop

River Trail

Blue Loop

Iron Bend Trail

river access

St. Johns River

N

0   0.1   0.2   0.3 mile

0   0.1   0.2   0.3 kilometer

Overview

As the St. Johns River snakes its way north from the Canaveral Marshes, it passes through a well-known series of vast wetlands and lakes: Lake Harney, Lake Jesup, and Lake Monroe. What you rarely see, however, unless you're a boater, are the connections between the lakes and marshes. Protecting 150 acres along a scenic stretch of the St. Johns River, Hickory Bluff Preserve showcases a rare natural river bluff along its trail system.

Route Details

Start at the kiosk, located in the shade near the exit to the parking area. Two loops make up the trail system. The blue-blazed River Trail, a mile long, goes out to the bluff and back. The red-blazed Pine Flatwoods Trail forms an extension for a longer loop back to the parking area. Leading into the pine flatwoods between dense walls of saw palmetto, the **River Trail** guides you past slash pines and sand live oaks. The trail is a pleasure to walk along, as the gatorbacks, or saw palmetto roots, have been removed and mulch covers the sand. Reaching a T-intersection, the firm surface ends and there is no signage to guide you forward. Turn right and the footpath becomes soft sand underfoot. The habitat transitions to scrubby flatwoods, with less shade and lots of gallberry. Young oaks peek out from between the saw palmetto, while gopher apple tempts gopher tortoises.

Passing an interpretive sign titled FLORIDA'S PINES, which recounts the four major types of pines found here, you see the first trail markers along the hike. A trio of these pines—soft, fluffy sand pine; tall longleaf pine; and slash pine—stands just beyond the marker, past an unmarked side trail.

You reach the first intersection of the two loop trails after 0.3 mile. Continue straight ahead, passing a primitive bench on the left made of chunks of telephone pole. Just beyond the bench is a small depression marsh. The marshy spot quickly yields to scrub, with silk bay appearing along the long corridor of saw palmetto. At the next junction, continue straight ahead into a shady oak hammock. The trail emerges onto an old road. Turn right.

Within a few moments, you draw within sight of the St. Johns River. The path leads through a campfire circle to a low, gentle slope down to a beach along the river. Cabbage palms line the far side of the river, which remains blissfully undeveloped. Walking back up to the fire ring, hang a left past the portable toilet. Continue through the forest through the picnic pavilion and beyond it, where a rough trail leads past a blue trail marker toward benches along the river.

Now comes the surprise and delight of this hike: Hickory Bluff is a natural bluff. It's high enough to provide a sweeping view of the river, and unlike most bluffs on the St. Johns River, it is not a midden; you'll find no snail shells here. You can walk right down to the river's edge and look up at the bluff too. Exit via the sandy corridor leading away from the river, following the trail markers. The sand in the footpath is deep and churned up, perhaps by the horses that also use these trails. A second- or third-growth forest, or trees that seem less than 100 years old, surrounds you. Scattered live oaks anchor the landscape.

In an open spot at 0.7 mile, you find the next trail junction at a fork. Turn left, following the blue marker. A stand of big, beautiful prickly pear cacti show off their blooms, if you are here in summer, and next to them is the namesake of the park, hickory trees. Behind you is an interpretive sign for a gopher tortoise and, just beyond it, a tortoise burrow with active trails leading out of it. A bench sits in the shade of an oak with a spray of goldfoot fern emerging from a crook in the trunk. The trail enters a broad tunnel shaded by sand live oaks and rusty lyonia. Leaves crunch beneath your feet.

Emerging from the shade, you pass a bench. At the next four-way junction of trails, the two loop trails meet again. Continue straight ahead to start the red-blazed **Pine Flatwoods Trail.** Meandering through the dense hardwood forest, the broad path is edged with bracken fern. Pinecones cover the footpath, and you can see some buildings off to the left. At 1 mile, you reach a four-way intersection.

A house is off to the left, beyond the preserve boundary fence. The red marker points you straight ahead past the bench and into the heart of the pine flatwoods, with a younger, denser forest of longleaf pines off to the right. Patches of bracken fern grow between the saw palmetto.

Bog buttons grow in the footpath as you pass another bench at 1.2 miles. The trail marker here, at the T-intersection, guides you to the right into scrubby flatwoods. There are taller pines in the distance, which offer some shade along a high wall of saw palmetto. When you reach the orange gate, you've completed the route. Walk around the gate and turn right to head back down to the kiosk where you started, wrapping up this 1.5-mile hike.

Nearby Attractions

Wiregrass Prairie Preserve (Hike 10, page 76) is east off Osteen-Maytown Road. Along FL 415, south of New Smyrna Boulevard in Osteen, the Osteen Diner is a colorful restaurant with a chicken coop in the parking lot and fresh veggies served up from local farms. Live folk music and homemade pies complement the dinner menu; visit **osteendiner.com.**

Directions

From I-4, Exit 108, drive east on DeBary Avenue; after 1.9 miles, it crosses Providence Road and becomes Doyle Avenue. Continue 5.9 miles to FL 415. Turn right. Make the third left onto New Smyrna Boulevard. Turn immediately left on Florida Avenue/Osteen-Maytown Road. Follow it through the small village of Osteen and continue 2.7 miles to Guise Road. Turn right and drive 1 mile. The trailhead is on the right.

5 Lake Harney Wilderness Area

SCENERY: ★ ★ ★ ★ ★
TRAIL CONDITION: ★ ★ ★ ★
CHILDREN: ★ ★ ★ ★
DIFFICULTY: ★ ★
SOLITUDE: ★ ★ ★

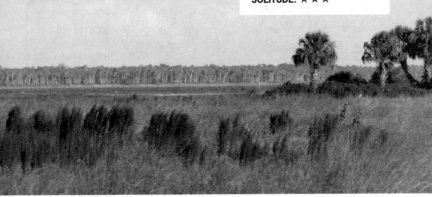

WILDFLOWERS IN THE FLOODPLAIN OF LAKE HARNEY

GPS TRAILHEAD COORDINATES: N28° 47.274' W81° 04.027'

DISTANCE & CONFIGURATION: 2.4 miles in a loop and a balloon

HIKING TIME: 1.5 hours

HIGHLIGHTS: Panoramic view of Lake Harney and the St. Johns River, a ghost town, ancient middens, and eagles' nests

ACCESS: Free; open daily, sunrise–sunset

MAPS: USGS *Osceola*

FACILITIES: Picnic tables and numerous benches along the route

WHEELCHAIR ACCESS: None

COMMENTS: This is a terminus for the Flagler Trail, a north–south bicycle trail through the county. The Floodplain Loop and a portion of the River Loop will be impassable if the river is in flood stage. Leashed pets are welcome.

CONTACTS: Seminole County Natural Lands Program (407) 665-2001; **seminolecountyfl .gov/parksrec/naturallands/harney.aspx**

Overview

One of the many Central Florida lakes formed by the St. Johns River as it travels north, Lake Harney outflows into a diverse, 300-acre preserve—the Lake Harney Wilderness Area. Deer browse in the uplands, and eagles nest in the tall pines. Ancient live oaks lead to the remains of the once-thriving lumber mill town of Osceola. A tall Timucua midden forms a lookout over the cypress-lined river. In the lowlands, acres of colorful wildflowers frame a picture-perfect panorama anchored by this pristine lake. Two loops totaling 2.4 miles provide a gentle walk through this beauty spot.

Route Details

From the parking area, walk to the far fence line opposite the entrance to the trailhead. Past a large southern magnolia, you'll find a gap through the fence to the **Floodplain Trail,** blazed with orange discs. As the name suggests, this loop heads into the floodplain of Lake Harney, so if the St. Johns River is in flood stage, it may be impassable. When the river is not in flood stage, the trail ushers you into a shady hammock of oaks, their limbs knitted overhead to form an unbroken canopy, with streamers of Spanish moss catching the sun and an opening ahead that showcases the lake.

The broad trail drops down rapidly through a stand of sweetgum trees. Flanked by tall cabbage palms and cypresses, the trail becomes a mowed path with seasonal wildflowers on either side. As you catch your first glimpse of Lake Harney, you will enjoy a big "wow" moment. The colors of the wildflowers in the foreground differ depending on the time of year. In summer, tall masses of coreopsis, our state flower and also known as tickseed, rise between the prairie grasses, painting the landscape in flecks of yellow. During the fall, sea myrtle bursts into fluffy white blooms, attracting colorful butterflies such as the tiger swallowtail. The far shoreline is outlined by a ridge of cabbage palms in tight rows, with cypresses rising behind them. Islands topped with cabbage palms lie in the middle of this

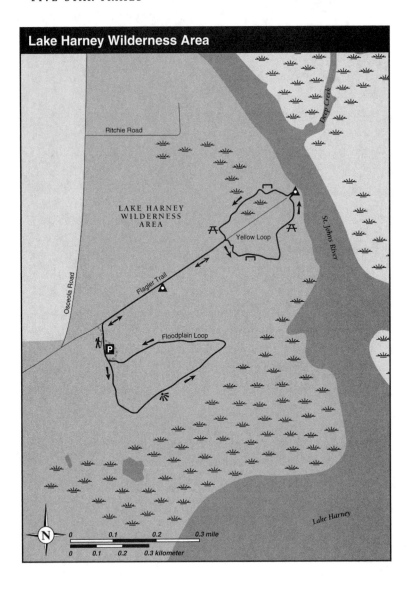

Lake Harney Wilderness Area

vast prairie. Depending on the lake level, the ribbon of water may be almost indiscernible in the distance. The trail makes a sharp left turn to follow the shoreline, paralleling the forest edge, a collection of cabbage palms, cedars, and pond cypresses on slightly higher ground. If you hear a distant buzz on the lake, it's from airboats, which can navigate its waters no matter how low they drop.

When the trail makes a sharp left to return to the shoreline, you may observe ibis and cattle egrets winging their way overhead to roost in the cypress as you take in a final sweeping view of this wildflower-dotted prairie. An orange fencepost marker confirms your route along a causeway bordered by a small canal. Partially shaded by oaks and cypresses, this long straightaway continues under a power line. You pass a wetlands pond as the trail returns to the parking area, completing the loop after 0.8 mile.

Walk across the parking area to the entrance side past a historical marker to the preserve's kiosk. Turn right under the park sign. Following the **Flagler Trail**, you're walking along the route of the Florida East Coast Railroad, circa 1911. Passionflower blooms beneath the pines that shade this section of trail. Traveling between two fenced-off pastures with paralleling power lines, you pass a mile marker for the Flagler Trail. Look up into the tall pines on the right, and you may spot an eagle's nest: This is where the birds are active during the spring and summer months as they raise their young. Eyes back on the trail, you will see that it is a broad, long, straight corridor. Oaks and pines close in, creating a shady canopy.

Keep alert for the yellow markers of the **River Loop** at 1.3 miles, and turn right. A tangle of oak limbs swaddled in resurrection fern frames a large pasture where deer may be grazing. The trail makes a sharp left and tunnels into the deep shade of the forest. It pops out under the power line with the St. Johns River off to the right. Making a sharp left, it follows the power-line easement past picnic tables in the shade of a live oak.

As the trail makes a curve, you're standing atop a large midden that creates a high bluff above the St. Johns River. Imagine a

Seminole village here. This is where Emaltha and his son Coacoochee, respected tribal leaders, established a settlement known to the U.S. Army as King Philip's Old Town and used it as a base for raids against military spreading into the area. Emaltha, outspoken against the forced removal of the Seminoles from Florida, was captured by U.S. Army forces in late 1837.

Turn right and climb up to the observation deck. It sits atop the midden and provides a nice view up the river. This was where the historic railroad crossed the river. As you leave this high spot, look straight ahead: the Flagler Trail makes a beeline back to the parking area. Turn right to stay on the yellow-blazed River Loop. At 1.7 miles, a brown sign marks the location of Osceola, the ghost town along the river. A thriving company town between 1916 and 1940, it centered on the timber mill run by the Osceola Cypress Company, which cut nearly 60,000 board feet of lumber each day. In its time, it was the biggest industrial complex in the county. But as the bald cypress was logged out, there was nothing left to process. Abandoned with the closure of the mill, the site was a fish camp prior to being protected by this preserve.

As you walk along, you'll skirt around an obvious foundation where the lumber mill once stood. The trail makes a sharp left, heading back into the forest at a bench under the shade of the moss-laden oaks. Walking beneath these ancient trees, look for foundations and other man-made right angles in the forest. Homes for 200 people once lined streets along the path you now walk. The trail makes another left and narrows down.

Picnic tables sit in the shade of a large live oak as the trail turns left again to complete the loop at 1.9 miles. Turn right and follow the **Flagler Trail** back out of the woods into the pastures, passing the eagle's nest again. At the trailhead entrance, turn left to walk to the parking area, completing the hike after 2.4 miles.

Nearby Attractions

The nearby town of Geneva is one of the best places in Florida to watch an old-fashioned Fourth of July parade—always on July 4. Festivities center around the Geneva Historical Museum on First Street. Bring your lawn chairs!

Directions

From the intersection of FL 46 and FL 415 east of Sanford, drive east on FL 46 toward Geneva for 2.8 miles. Turn left on West Osceola Road. The road becomes Osceola Fish Camp Road after 7.6 miles. The large parking area is on the right after another 0.7 mile. Both trails are accessed through the parking area, which also serves as a trail-head for the Flagler Trail, a cross-county bicycle route that bisects this wilderness area.

6

Lake Jesup
Conservation Area:
East Tract

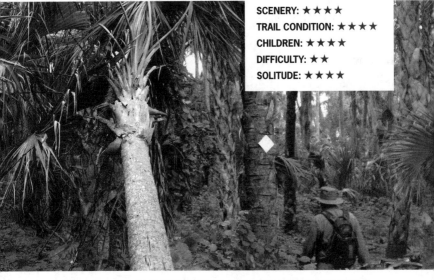

SCENERY: ★ ★ ★ ★
TRAIL CONDITION: ★ ★ ★ ★
CHILDREN: ★ ★ ★ ★
DIFFICULTY: ★ ★
SOLITUDE: ★ ★ ★ ★

HIKING INTO THE PALM HAMMOCK AT LAKE JESUP CONSERVATION AREA

GPS TRAILHEAD COORDINATES: N28° 43.006' W81° 11.285'

DISTANCE & CONFIGURATION: 2.1-mile balloon

HIKING TIME: 1.5 hours

HIGHLIGHTS: Observation tower with view of Lake Jesup, dry palm hammocks

ACCESS: Free; open daily, sunrise–sunset

MAPS: USGS *Oviedo*; sjrwmd.com/trailguides/pdfs/lakejesup_easttrail.pdf

FACILITIES: None

WHEELCHAIR ACCESS: None

COMMENTS: Parking is limited. Leashed pets welcome. Loop may flood when the
St. Johns River is high.

CONTACTS: Lake Jesup Conservation Area, St. Johns River Water Management District
(386) 329-4404; sjrwmd.com/recreationguide/lakejesup

Overview

With more than 5,200 acres along the shores of Lake Jesup—a shallow, expansive waterway fed by the St. Johns River—Lake Jesup Conservation Area encompasses vast floodplain prairies that dip beneath the lake's level as it rises. On the east side of the lake, in rural Black Hammock, the East Tract offers the only observation tower along Lake Jesup's shores. It's an easy walk through forests of oaks and palms on dry land to enjoy this bird's-eye view of the lake. Due to weekend boat traffic, however, it is best experienced on weekdays.

Route Details

From the trailhead, walk toward the trail kiosk set under the oaks across a small stretch of pasture. The footpath enters the cool shade of the first oak hammock, paralleling Elm Street for a short distance. Making a sharp right, the trail continues toward taller oaks draped in Spanish moss and rounds a curve to the left. The trail tacks back and forth between oak hammocks and former pasture, crossing two small footbridges over ephemeral streams. Emerging at the remains of an old campsite, it drops through a swale and arrives at a T-intersection. Turn right. After 0.5 mile, you arrive at the T-intersection with the loop portion of the trail.

Forming a boundary between a restored slash pine forest in an old pasture and a dense hammock of cedars, live oaks, and cabbage palms, the trail follows an old forest road with scattered pine duff underfoot. Vegetation leans in from both sides, creating a tunnel of shade. Passing a hydrologic data collection site in an open area framed by cabbage palms, you reach a faint fork in the trail. Keep left. You may hear the buzz of airboats as the trail drops down into the lush lakeside hammock of tall cabbage palms and ancient live oaks. Bromeliads dangle everywhere, perched on tree limbs, clinging to leaves, hanging from grapevines, even caught in streamers of Spanish moss. Tossed from the forest canopy during high winds, many thickly carpet the forest floor.

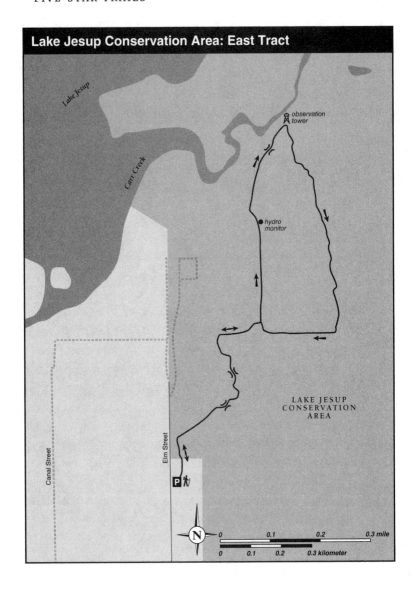

Lake Jesup Conservation Area: East Tract

Lake Jesup

Carr Creek

observation
tower

hydro
monitor

LAKE JESUP
CONSERVATION
AREA

Canal Street

Elm Street

N

| 0 | 0.1 | 0.2 | 0.3 mile |

| 0 | 0.1 | 0.2 | 0.3 kilometer |

The deeper you descend into the forest, the grander it becomes. A slight aroma of orange blossoms wafts on the breeze, as does the smell of freshwater as the trail draws closer to the lake. Reaching a natural drainage that feeds into Lake Jesup, you cross a footbridge with a view of the marshes. Curving left, the trail continues toward the lake.

After 1 mile, you reach the big observation tower. It's a sturdy wooden structure tucked into the oak and palm hammock and is adjoined by a hitching post for equestrians. Climb to the top for the panorama. The tower faces north, toward Davis Point, up the narrower portion of the lake that connects to the main flow of the St. Johns River. Marshes dotted with cabbage palms line the far shores and rim the islands in the lake. White ibis and cattle egrets wing across the water in large flocks. Fishing boats bob in the shallows. If it's a clear day, you may be able to see the control tower at the Sanford International Airport at the horizon line to the northwest.

As you leave the tower, turn left. Look for white diamond markers on the cabbage palm trunks. These mark the return route. Ditched and diked for agriculture more than a century ago, this part of the trail remains high and dry most of the year. After a short stretch of finding your way between the palm trunks, the trail widens and becomes obvious. The footpath undulates over old plow lines, the legacy of agriculture along the lake creating rugged terrain. You pass several fallen oaks, their trunks covered in mosses, the intricate intertwining of weathered roots interlaced with the green ribbons of sword ferns. Cabbage palms crowd in very closely, creating a tunnel of fronds overhead.

After 1.4 miles you cross a causeway over a culvert for a deep ditch filled with prehistoric-looking giant leather ferns. The trail turns right to parallel the ditch on a berm, the dark water within covered with a smattering of water spangles, floating ferns that glisten in the sun. Turning a corner to the right, the trail completes the loop after 1.6 miles. Turn left. Keep alert as you pop out of the tunnel of oaks for a double diamond marker on a post. Turn left. The trail

57

immediately drops through a swale and passes back through the old campsite. Watch for the white diamonds along the well-trodden footpath to find your way back as the trail slips back and forth between oak hammocks and open spaces, crossing two footbridges on the way back to the trailhead.

Nearby Attractions

Don't miss Black Hammock Adventures! In addition to an excellent restaurant, this funky waterfront fish camp offers airboat rides that take you across Lake Jesup to see the alligators and the islands: **theblackhammock.com.** Black Hammock Wilderness Area (Hike 1, page 26) is just up the road.

Directions

From FL 417, Exit 44, follow FL 434 toward Oviedo. After 1 mile, turn left at the Black Hammock sign on the curve onto DeLeon Street. Continue down DeLeon Street to a T at Howard Street. Turn right onto Howard Street and follow it for 1.2 miles to Elm Street. Turn left. Continue another 1.2 miles to the trailhead entrance on the right.

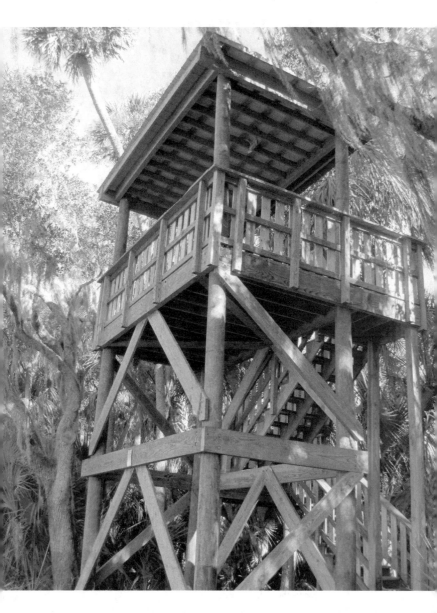

OBSERVATION TOWER OVERLOOKING LAKE JESUP

7

Lake Monroe Conservation Area: Kratzert Tract

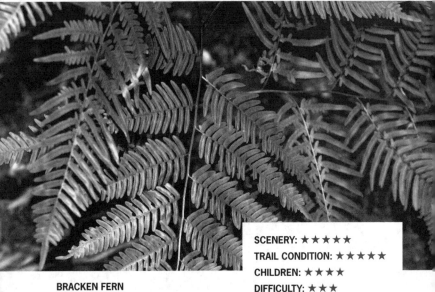

BRACKEN FERN

SCENERY: ★ ★ ★ ★ ★
TRAIL CONDITION: ★ ★ ★ ★ ★
CHILDREN: ★ ★ ★ ★
DIFFICULTY: ★ ★
SOLITUDE: ★ ★ ★

GPS TRAILHEAD COORDINATES: N28° 49.919' W81° 11.486'

DISTANCE & CONFIGURATION: 1.5-mile loop

HIKING TIME: 45 minutes

HIGHLIGHTS: Ancient oaks and palms

ACCESS: Free; open daily, sunrise–sunset

MAPS: USGS *Osteen*

FACILITIES: None

WHEELCHAIR ACCESS: None

COMMENTS: Leashed pets permitted. This trail will flood when the St. Johns River is in flood stage. The conservation area is seasonally open for hunting; please check ahead for hunt dates at **myfwc.com/viewing/recreation/wmas /cooperative/lake-monroe**.

CONTACTS: St. Johns River Water Management District (386) 329-4404; **floridaswater .com/recreationguide/lakemonroe**

Overview

For a quick dip into the beauty of the St. Johns River floodplain, the Kratzert White Loop offers a family-friendly walk beneath ancient oaks and cabbage palms of enormous size. The 1.5-mile loop is well maintained and easy to follow. It's especially fun with kids, who will enjoy the long stretches of narrow, mazelike corridors through dense, tall saw palmettos. Plus there are bridges to cross and gopher tortoise burrows in obvious spots. If you're looking for a short but gorgeous hike, this trek on the east shore of the St. Johns River fills the bill.

Route Details

After a look at the kiosk, turn right to walk the trail counterclockwise, following the footpath into a restored longleaf pine forest on former ranchland. Winged sumac and wild persimmon peep out of the understory. The path is grassy, mown, and obvious, but white blazes do confirm the route. After 0.25 mile, you dip through a small floodplain lined with young sweetgum trees and large wax myrtle. As the trail rises up again, you can see the vast floodplain forest off to your left beyond the pines. Reed Ellis Road is close enough to see and hear off to the right, but the trail quickly turns away from the road into a patch of open scrub on the edge of the floodplain. Dropping down to the right under live oaks and palms, you pass a patch of coreopsis, our state flower, which is often in bloom. Turning left and away from the wildflowers, you're in a hardwood hammock with clumps of saw palmetto through the understory, oaks forming a canopy above. A wide bridge, proudly inscribed as an Eagle Scout project, crosses an ephemeral waterway at the 0.5-mile mark. The trail rises through another pasture planted in longleaf pine. Raspberry bushes poke through the tall grass, and paw-paw shows off ivory-colored blooms in winter. It's slippery underfoot, between the grass and the pine needles. There are several gopher tortoise burrows right along the footpath.

Heading downhill, you enter a shady forest of oaks, saw palmetto, and large longleaf pines, where beds of sword fern crowd the

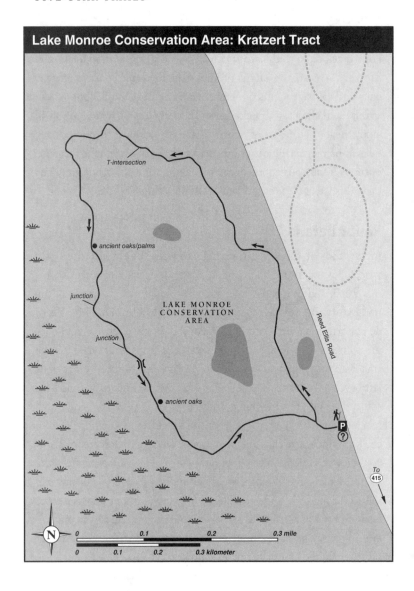

Lake Monroe Conservation Area: Kratzert Tract

T-intersection

ancient oaks/palms

junction

LAKE MONROE
CONSERVATION
AREA

junction

ancient oaks

Reed Ellis Road

To
415

N

| 0 | 0.1 | 0.2 | 0.3 mile |

| 0 | 0.1 | 0.2 | 0.3 kilometer |

footpath as it parallels the meandering route of a sand-bottomed stream. Roots jut out into the trail, and the oaks around you are much larger. Off to the left, you can see the pines through a window in the dense hammock. At a T-intersection with an unmarked trail, turn right. A jog to the left propels you uphill through a tangle of saw palmetto beneath a corridor of southern magnolia. The trail twists and turns down a narrow corridor, emerging in another stand of southern magnolia before plunging into the twisting, winding path again. At 0.7 mile, the trail rises up under tall oaks laden with bromeliads, many dangling from grapevines, the canopy well overhead. It then drops back down into the palmetto maze before winding beneath cabbage palms of regal stature, palms that rise more than 100 feet above the forest floor. The air is humid, and every tree sports colonies of bromeliads and orchids. Look overhead for dense mats of resurrection fern; fine sprays of wild pine; the purple, red, and yellow spikes of cardinal wild pine; and grasslike giant blades of greenfly orchids nestled in the crooks of tree limbs.

The trail jogs right through the thickets of saw palmetto as you continue under the grand oak canopy. You pass between two cabbage palm trunks before the corridor gets much denser with young trees. At 1 mile, you reach a trail junction. Follow the white blazes left. The elevation slowly rises, leading you beneath laurel oaks and water oaks. At the next trail junction, continue straight ahead. A lazy waterway meanders off to the right as it makes its way down to the St. Johns River, its banks lined with netted chain fern. The trail crosses a bridge before it broadens considerably, passing through another old palm hammock. You walk under a massive live oak that looks just plain furry from the amount of resurrection fern and bromeliads swaddling its limbs. A cabbage palm grows right through the crook of the tree.

As the trail slowly climbs out of the shady hammock, it rises through stands of tall saw palmetto, emerging again at the pine forest at 1.3 miles. Follow the footpath along the ecotone. As you come over a rise, you see the trailhead kiosk and parking lot, completing the 1.5-mile loop.

Nearby Attractions

Historic downtown Sanford features art galleries, antiques shops, and street festivals. Walk more than a mile along the waterfront on the RiverWalk, with a large playground and splash area the kids will love: **sanfordfl.gov.** At the Central Florida Zoo, more than 400 animals live within the riverfront forest; explore the treetops above them in the ZOOm Air Adventure Park: **centralfloridazoo.org.**

Directions

From I-4, Exit 101, Sanford, head east on FL 46 for 3.8 miles to US 17-92, crossing into the downtown district. Continue through the historic downtown for 1.1 miles to Mellonville Avenue. Turn right and drive 0.7 mile to County Road 415 (Celery Avenue). Turn left. Follow CR 415 for 2.8 miles to FL 415. Turn left and cross the St. Johns River Bridge, driving 2.4 miles to Reed Ellis Road. Make a left and continue 0.9 mile, passing the Lake Monroe Conservation Area parking area, to the second parking corral on the left.

Lyonia Preserve

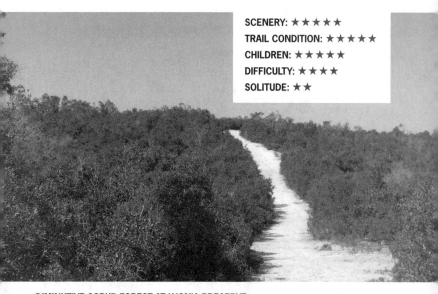

SCENERY: ★ ★ ★ ★
TRAIL CONDITION: ★ ★ ★ ★
CHILDREN: ★ ★ ★ ★
DIFFICULTY: ★ ★ ★
SOLITUDE: ★ ★

DIMINUTIVE SCRUB FOREST AT LYONIA PRESERVE

GPS TRAILHEAD COORDINATES: N28° 55.813' W81° 13.527'

DISTANCE & CONFIGURATION: 2.3-mile triple loops

HIKING TIME: 1.5 hours

HIGHLIGHTS: Interactions with Florida scrub-jays, detailed interpretive information, views from high ridges

ACCESS: Free; open daily, sunrise–sunset

MAPS: USGS *Lake Helen*; **lyoniapreserve.com/lyonia1.htm**

FACILITIES: Nature center with gift shop, café, restrooms, and regularly scheduled interpretive programs

WHEELCHAIR ACCESS: None

COMMENTS: Pets not permitted. Do not feed the scrub-jays. An interpretive guide, keyed to markers in the preserve, is available at the environmental center.

CONTACTS: Lyonia Preserve (386) 789-7207 and **lyoniapreserve.com**; Volusia County Government Land Acquisition and Management (386) 424-6834 and **volusia.org/growth/lyonia.htm**

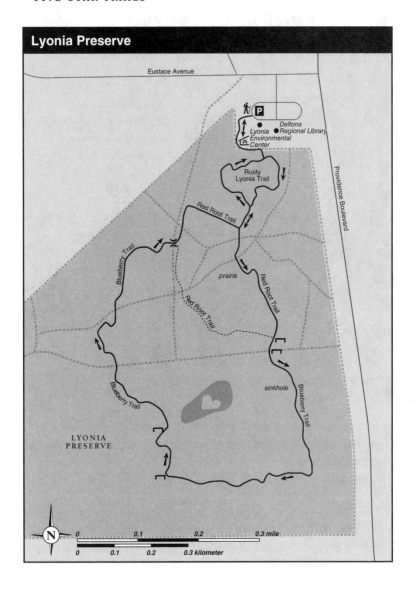

Lyonia Preserve

Eustace Avenue

Deltona
Lyonia Regional Library
Environmental
Center

Rusty
Lyonia Trail

Red Root Trail

Blueberry Trail

prairie

Red Root Trail

Red Root Trail

sinkhole

Blueberry Trail

Blueberry Trail

LYONIA
PRESERVE

Providence Boulevard

N

0   0.1   0.2   0.3 mile

0   0.1   0.2   0.3 kilometer

Overview

The Florida scrub-jay is a colorful, large bird, noticeable as it flies past in a streak of white and blue. It is Florida's only endemic bird, found nowhere else in the world. At Lyonia Preserve, you'll see them up close, and this is the best place in Florida to photograph these otherwise rare birds. The trail system traverses challenging scrub terrain with high hills and little shade, but the habitats are beautiful, and the delight of interacting with scrub-jays makes this a must-visit for the entire family.

Route Details

With its trailhead adjacent to the outdoor amphitheater at the Lyonia Environmental Center, the entrance trail guides you downhill through an interpretive corridor of common plants of the scrub habitat, such as shiny blueberry and myrtle oak. Pass through the picnic pavilion, which has a map of the trail, and turn left along the fence line. Make the first right at the beaten path into the diminutive forest. The series of three stacked loops begins here with the **Rusty Lyonia Trail,** the gentlest of the loops. Because of the configuration of the trail system, you can tailor your hike to the time and stamina of your group.

Turn right at the trail junction for a slow, steady descent through the tiny trees. Florida scrub-jays require the naturally stunted oaks found in a young scrub forest, as they gather and bury acorns as part of their diet and nest low to the ground. Look for the scrub palmetto, found only in this habitat. Although it looks like a small saw palmetto, the leaf stem extends into the frond, unlike saw palmetto. The scrub-jays pull fibers from this palm to build their nests. Rounding a corner, the trail continues down a straight corridor before turning left and downhill. At an intersection with an orange marker, continue straight ahead.

On the next downhill, the trail offers a view across to the next ridge. This 360-acre preserve of ancient sand dunes is the highest ground in Volusia County, rising up to 75 feet above sea level. At 0.3 mile, this trail completes its loop, rejoining the main route. Turn right. Within a few moments, you reach the beginning of the **Red Root Trail,** the central trail of the system. Continue straight ahead at the trail junction. Florida rosemary grows in dense clusters amid the bright white sand of the open scrub. One lone pine stands tall over the trail on the edge of a wet prairie, which is ringed with a gradient of colorful grasses. As the trail turns away from the prairie, it heads uphill, winding its way under large oak trees.

Atop the hills, you start to hear the chatter of scrub-jays back and forth to each other. They travel in family groups, one serving as a sentinel to warn the others of danger. An unmarked trail comes in from the right at a bench. Look up, and you may see a scrub-jay perched in the nearby oak. When you reach the blue markers and a bench at 0.7 mile, you're at the junction for the longest loop, the **Blueberry Trail.** To stay on the outer circuit around the preserve, continue straight. From the next promontory, there is a great view across the scrub ridges. The trail descends toward tall longleaf pines that surround a sinkhole. As the trail climbs uphill again, notice the desert-like surroundings. The scrub is Florida's version of desert, with poor soil and little surface water, its plants adapted to heat and dryness.

Rounding a curve, look off to your right to see a sweep of white across the ancient dunes in the distance. Despite the sand, the footpath is hard-packed as you ascend the hills. As the trail drops down and rises back up, you see a copse of oaks on a summit. Reaching that summit, you savor the merest puddle of shade before the trail rounds another corner, continuing up and over more ridges toward the high point. Tucked off the footpath, a bench at 1.2 miles provides a panoramic view of the preserve and a vast wetland below from this promontory, 50 feet above sea level.

Dropping down a steep slope of white sand to curve past the wet prairie, the trail follows the prairie's edge past a bench. Sandhill cranes frequent the prairie and a family of scrub-jays lives near its edge. As the trail turns away from the prairie, it continues up a straightaway and curves right, starting another ascent through the diminutive trees. A cross-trail provides scenic views on both sides before the trail enters a much denser part of the sand pine forest. A patch of rosemary scrub flanks the trail before you reach a brief tunnel of shade. Ascending the next ridge, the trail crosses a sand road next to a bench. Scrub-jay chatter becomes more intense. Over the next 0.5 mile, it's likely you'll encounter many of them, thus the lengthy estimate of hiking time. You don't want to rush past the birds as they peck at acorns, peer down from branches, and sometimes even hop on your head.

After a sweeping arc to the right and downhill, you reach the end of the **Blueberry Trail,** just past a firebreak, meeting the **Red Root Trail** at 1.8 miles. Although the arrow points to the right, turn left to stay on the outer loop. The sand becomes softer underfoot as you cross a sand road. After the next descent and ascent, you reach a bench where scrub-jays often appear. The trail makes a hard right down a shady corridor, descending to the end of the **Red Root Trail.** Turn left. When you reach the orange-blazed **Rusty Lyonia Trail,** turn right. You emerge at the fence behind the environmental center. Turn left and follow the trail back through the picnic pavilion to exit, completing the 2.3-mile hike.

Nearby Attractions

The Lyonia Environmental Center offers hands-on activities for kids to learn about scrub habitat, the watershed, and the animals of the scrub: **lyoniapreserve.com/lec.htm.** For a full day of wildlife-watching, combine this hike with a visit to Blue Spring State Park (Hikes 28 and 29, pages 184 and 189), the best place in Florida to see manatees during the winter months: **floridastateparks.org/bluespring.**

Directions

Take I-4, Exit 54, Deltona, to Howland Boulevard (FL 472). Drive 2.2 miles south. Turn right on Providence Boulevard and continue 0.7 mile. Turn right on Eustace Avenue. The entrance is immediately on the left. The Deltona Public Library and the Lyonia Environmental Center share the parking area.

9

Spring Hammock Preserve

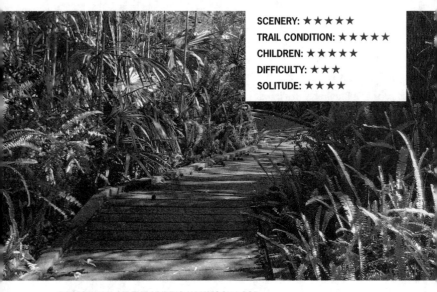

SCENERY: ★ ★ ★ ★ ★
TRAIL CONDITION: ★ ★ ★ ★ ★
CHILDREN: ★ ★ ★ ★ ★
DIFFICULTY: ★ ★
SOLITUDE: ★ ★ ★

BOARDWALK ON THE HYDRIC HAMMOCK LOOP

GPS TRAILHEAD COORDINATES: N28° 43.302' W81° 18.424'

DISTANCE & CONFIGURATION: 3.1-mile loop and spur

HIKING TIME: 2 hours

HIGHLIGHTS: Massive, ancient cypress trees

ACCESS: Free; open daily, sunrise–sunset

MAPS: USGS *Casselberry*

FACILITIES: Restrooms, picnic pavilions

WHEELCHAIR ACCESS: None

COMMENTS: Restrooms are open only on weekdays, when the Seminole County Environmental Studies Center hosts school groups. Active removal of invasive air potato plants means you'll see a lot of buckets along the trails to toss the potato-shaped tubers into, should you stumble across any in the footpath.

CONTACTS: Seminole County Natural Lands Program (407) 665-2001; **seminolecountyfl .gov/parksrec/naturallands/hammock.aspx; environmentalstudiescenter.org**

Overview

While it was painful to lose Florida's 3,500-year-old cypress tree, "The Senator," to a fire in early 2012, most visitors to this celebrated icon never realized that the Big Tree was just one of many ancient cypresses in the forests of Spring Hammock Preserve. Used as an environmental education center for local public schools, the trail system has dozens of possible routes using a mix of mazelike short, scenic trails; more adventuresome and difficult trails; the paved Cross Seminole Trail; and boardwalks through these shady glades along Lake Jesup. Home of the beloved Mud Walk, the first down-and-dirty outdoor experience for many area schoolchildren, Spring Hammock Preserve has hiking options for adventurers of every age.

Route Details

Starting beneath a canopy of pine trees on the **Pine Woods Trail**—one of many short, signposted trails within the preserve—walk through the picnic pavilion (a nice option for your lunch after the hike) and turn right on the **Azalea Trail,** walking through a dense hardwood hammock with many oaks and pines. The footpath can be mushy underfoot. As the Azalea Trail ends, turn right and go past the **Basswood Trail** to start walking down a boardwalk through a hydric hammock. It passes the **Smilax Trail** and a set of benches before ending. Continue past the **Primary Trail** and a second picnic pavilion to Sweetgum Circle, an outdoor classroom with benches circled beneath the trees. You can hear the hum of traffic on FL 419 as the trail scrambles up a small knoll separated from the highway by a ditch.

This is where the hike gets adventuresome. Dropping down through a stand of cabbage palms, the trail comes to a T-intersection. To the right is an old railroad trestle. In front of you is Soldier's Creek, a tannic waterway that winds down toward Lake Jesup. Turn left to follow it. At 0.25 mile, you pass a trail coming in from the left. Twisting and winding on the high sand banks above the creek, the trail provides good views of the waterway, which is deeply scoured into the

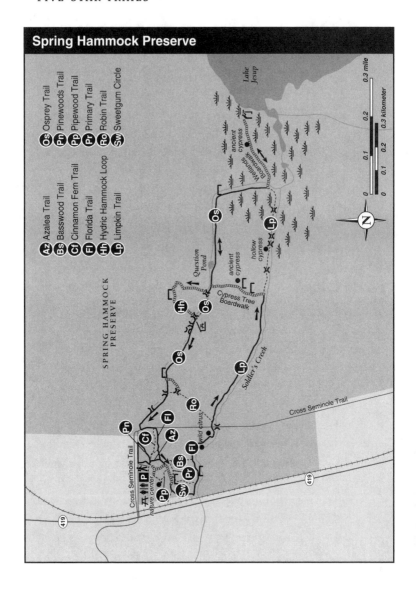

Spring Hammock Preserve

SPRING HAMMOCK PRESERVE

Az Azalea Trail
Bs Basswood Trail
Cf Cinnamon Fern Trail
Fl Florida Trail
Hh Hydric Hammock Loop
Lp Limpkin Trail

Os Osprey Trail
Pn Pinewoods Trail
Pp Pipewood Trail
Pr Primary Trail
Ro Robin Trail
Sw Sweetgum Circle

Lake Jesup

ancient cypress

Wetlands Boardwalk

Question Pond

ancient cypress

Cypress Tree Boardwalk

hollow cypress

Soldier's Creek

Cross Seminole Trail

wild citrus

Cross Seminole Trail

nature center

419

419

earth by rushes of water from upstream during strong rains. As you walk beneath deep shade, there are undercuts beneath the footpath from times of flooding. You pass two benches in quick succession, and another trail junction. Watch your footing, as the footpath is narrow and littered with fallen citrus as it winds between cypress knees.

After 0.4 mile, you emerge beneath open skies onto the **Cross Seminole Trail,** a bike path that runs the length of the county. Cross over it and continue straight ahead, crossing a log bridge. At the fork, keep right to walk the **Limpkin Trail,** which follows the creek. It's on an old tramway, slightly elevated over the water, used more than a century ago to remove the giant cypresses for timber. Fortunately, in the forests ahead of you there are still a handful of these ancient trees, each with a flaw that spared them from a sawmill. Working its way around a dark, shimmering swampy bay of shallow water atop dense muck, the trail is crowded by palm fronds. The footpath gets muckier as floodplain trees tower overhead, the sweetgums and maples sporting colorful leaves in winter. It may be necessary to wade the next short section of the trail if the creek is high, as it intrudes into the trail.

When you reach the boardwalk at 0.9 mile, it's an important decision point. When the creek is low, it's safe to continue straight ahead and parallel the creek to reach the boardwalk out to the giant cypress. You will still get your feet wet in places within the floodplain. But if you've already had to wade, don't even try to continue along the creek. To keep dry, turn left to make use of the boardwalk, which leads to the first massive cypress along this hike. A platform with a bench provides a viewing spot to stare up, up, up into its high branches. Looking down into the surrounding swamp, you'll see cinnamon ferns, royal ferns, and marsh ferns. Surrounding the one big cypress are many others of distinctive size.

The boardwalk ends at a T-intersection with an old forest road. Turn right. This road provides a backbone to the trail systems at this far end of the preserve, which reach deeper into the floodplain forests. Curving past Question Pond, a spring surrounded by cabbage palms, the trail reaches the boardwalk to Lake Jesup at 1.4 miles. Turn left.

Down this boardwalk, you walk beneath and between cypress trees of incredible size, some with bases as large as a small car, others with knees that are taller than you are. The crowns of these trees are easier to see in fall and winter when the leaves are off the surrounding trees. Scanning through the forest, you can see many more ancient cypresses in the distance. The boardwalk ends with a view of Lake Jesup. Turn around and retrace your steps back to the forest road, and make a right. You pass a bench and are back to Question Pond at 2.1 miles.

The **Hydric Hammock Trail** starts soon on the right. Crossing a small bridge to start this boardwalk, this is a tame trail intersected several times by the sloppy Mud Walk that the kids enjoy; you can see footprints in the muck at the trail crossings. Clusters of glossy dark-green needle palms crowd the boardwalk. These cold-hardy palms prefer this cooler, well-shaded habitat. The deeper you go into this swamp forest, the more mosquitoes you'll encounter. Sword ferns emerge in mounds from old cypress stumps.

When the trail deposits you back at the forest road, turn right. There are steps off to the left down to the waterway, where the kids assemble for the Mud Walk. You'll pass a pavilion on the left. At the next four-way junction, continue straight ahead to pass the far end of the Mud Walk. After you emerge at the intersection of the park road and the **Cross Seminole Trail,** turn left to walk briefly down the paved trail. Turn off to the right at an old sign that says **Florida Trail.** You're returning to uplands habitats, passing several tulip poplars that make up the southernmost stand of these trees in the United States. Crooked branches of rusty lyonia rise above the trail beneath the canopy of slash pines.

At the junction with the **Cinnamon Fern Trail,** continue straight ahead. This area can get boggy, and sometimes the bog bridges float right off the trail into the woods before they are put back again. Reaching the **Azalea Trail,** turn right, then left for the **Pine Woods Trail,** retracing your first few steps through the pavilion and back to your car after 3.1 miles.

Nearby Attractions

Biking the Cross Seminole Trail is a lot of fun, with the nearest easy-to-access trailhead across FL 419 at Soldier's Creek Park. North along US 17/92 in Sanford, the Central Florida Zoo and Botanical Gardens features zip lines through the trees above the wild creatures: **centralfloridazoo.org.** You're also just up the road from Travel Country Outdoors, the region's largest outfitter for hiking and paddle sports: **travelcountry.com.**

Directions

From I-4, Exit 98 (Lake Mary/Heathrow), drive east on Lake Mary Boulevard for 1.6 miles to Longwood–Lake Mary Road. Turn right and continue 2.5 miles to where it ends at Ronald Reagan Boulevard. Turn left and make the first right onto General Hutchinson Parkway. Continue to the traffic light at US 17/92. Turn left. After 0.8 mile, make a right at the light onto FL 419. Drive 0.6 mile to the preserve entrance, on the left across from the ball fields at Osprey Trail. Enter the gates and park on the right.

10

Wiregrass Prairie Preserve

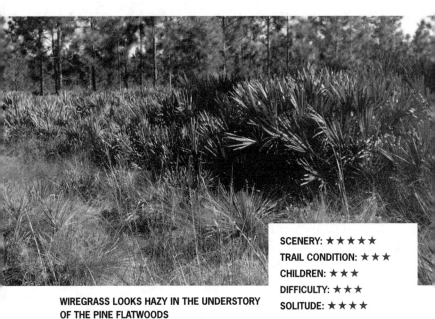

SCENERY: ★ ★ ★ ★ ★
TRAIL CONDITION: ★ ★ ★
CHILDREN: ★ ★ ★
DIFFICULTY: ★ ★ ★
SOLITUDE: ★ ★ ★ ★

WIREGRASS LOOKS HAZY IN THE UNDERSTORY
OF THE PINE FLATWOODS

GPS TRAILHEAD COORDINATES: N28° 54.329' W81° 03.167'

DISTANCE & CONFIGURATION: 3.3-mile balloon

HIKING TIME: 1.5 hours

HIGHLIGHTS: Expansive pine savanna, colorful wildflowers

ACCESS: Free; open daily, sunrise–sunset

MAPS: USGS *Lake Ashby*

FACILITIES: None

WHEELCHAIR ACCESS: None

COMMENTS: Trails are shared with off-road cyclists and equestrians. Leashed pets permitted. If the area is damp, the mosquitoes can be voracious.

CONTACTS: Volusia County Government Land Acquisition and Management (386) 424-6834; **volusia.org/growth/wiregrass.htm**

Overview

Part of a 1,400-acre watershed encompassing wetlands that flow out of Lake Ashby toward the St. Johns River basin, Wiregrass Prairie Preserve is a wild and rugged place in a distinctly rural setting. This hike explores the Yellow Loop, the southernmost of the three loops within the preserve and the only one with a trailhead accessible by passenger car. It guides you into the namesake of the preserve, a pine savanna with an extensive wiregrass prairie, one of the showiest habitats in the region.

Route Details

Starting from the map kiosk at the parking area, follow the yellow markers down an elevated grassy berm. This long straightaway follows a fence line with an adjacent ranch. Rest assured this is not the scenic part of the trail but a necessary connector to lead you to the loop. Making a gentle left away from the fence, the trail enters former pastureland replanted with longleaf pine. Goldenrod lines both sides of the footpath, and you see cypress domes off to the right.

You come to the intersection with the loop portion of the trail at a bench after 0.6 mile. Turn right. The trail continues to parallel the fence. Crossing a stream that runs through a culvert, you see pine flatwoods off to the left, high and dry, with an understory of saw palmetto. Ranchland, open pine savanna with cypress domes, stretches off to the right. This is classic Central Florida cattle country, grassy and flat, with clumps of saw palmetto and longleaf pines.

The trail makes a sharp left away from the fence. Soon after, an eye-catching display of silvery-blue-tinged saw palmetto stands out among the standard green variety. At 1.2 miles, you leave the berm and enter the prairie, an expanse of longleaf pine savanna to the left. The wall of trees on the right is a bayhead swamp delineating the edge of the savanna. Making a sharp bend to the left, the trail immerses you in the prairie's wide-open spaces, dense with wiregrass, the namesake of the preserve. Yellow stargrass adds a hint of

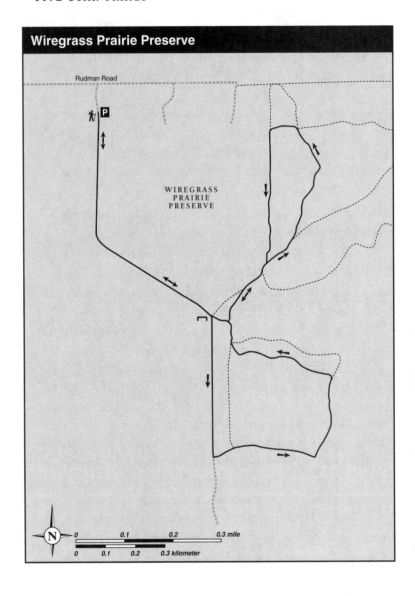

Wiregrass Prairie Preserve

Rudman Road

WIREGRASS
PRAIRIE
PRESERVE

N

0   0.1   0.2   0.3 mile

0   0.1   0.2   0.3 kilometer

color to the landscape, along with fleabane and the feathery arcs of blazing star, which blooms in a showy display each fall.

Around 1.5 miles, a stand of pond pines grows near the bay-head, distinctive with its tousled-looking needles, some protruding from the trunks themselves. There are also excellent examples of the different stages of longleaf pine: grass, when it can be mistaken for wiregrass; candle, when it shoots up quickly and starts sprouting branches; and full-grown of various sizes. You pass a gopher tortoise burrow just as the trail swings right, leaving the prairie behind for denser pine flatwoods.

At the T-intersection, take the trail to the right, following the marker. If it rained recently, you may encounter soggy spots in the footpath, some ankle-deep in places. Entering a denser, older pine savanna, the trail comes up to the next junction at 1.6 miles. Passing an unmarked trail on the left, continue straight ahead. The trail splits around a clump of saw palmetto, where an arrow encourages you to keep right. The next junction defines the upper loop in the trail system. Turn right. A line of cypresses marks the horizon as you emerge into another pine savanna. Keep left, and the prairie opens up again around you, providing sweeping views across a grand and beautiful landscape. As the trail curves to the left, it offers even better views. The saw palmetto is short, only 1 or 2 feet high, so as you cross this panoramic landscape, you can see trail markers in the distance.

At 2.2 miles, you reach a trail junction. Turn left to leave the prairie, heading for the tree line. This portion of the trail is a bit rougher than the rest, with deer tracks leading through muddy spots. Turn left at the T-intersection, where you may find the bright-pink wildflower sabatia in bloom. The trail follows the fence, with a view to the left of the prairie that you just crossed. Stay to the left at the next fork. It can be wet underfoot where a cypress dome drains across the trail beneath the longleaf pines. Keep watching for the next marker as you work your way through this patchwork of puddles.

Passing a trail coming in from the left at another drainage area, you complete the upper loop after 2.6 miles. Rejoining the main trail,

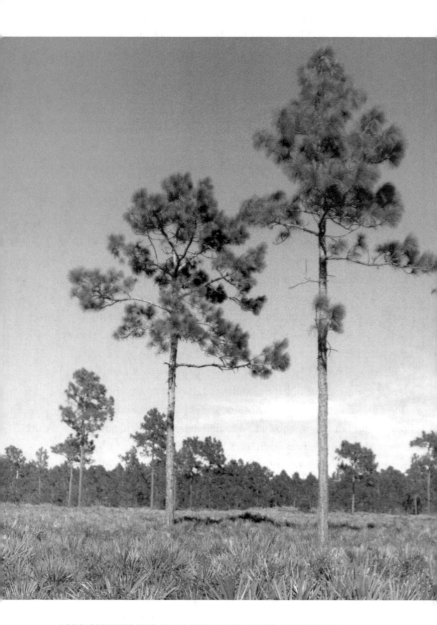

LONGLEAF PINES RISE ABOVE THE SAW PALMETTO UNDERSTORY

watch for the second turn to the right, which is blazed with orange markers. Dog fennel grows tall between the pines and the saw palmetto along this short corridor, which emerges at the first junction with a bench, completing the overall loop. Continue straight ahead, following the grassy berm you came in on, to complete the hike after 3.3 miles.

Nearby Attractions

Hickory Bluff Preserve (Hike 4, page 43) is west off Osteen-Maytown Road. Along FL 415 south of New Smyrna Boulevard in Osteen, the Osteen Diner is a colorful restaurant with a chicken coop in the parking lot and fresh veggies served up from local farms. Live folk music and homemade pies complement the dinner menu: **osteendiner.com.**

Directions

From I-4, Exit 108, drive east on DeBary Avenue; after 1.9 miles, it crosses Providence Road and becomes Doyle Avenue. Continue 5.9 miles to FL 415. Turn right. Make the third left onto New Smyrna Boulevard. Turn immediately left on Florida Avenue/Osteen-Maytown Road. Follow it through the small village of Osteen. Continue 5.7 miles to Pell Road. Turn left. Follow Pell Road for 4.1 miles. It becomes a dirt road and passes a fire tower. Turn right onto Rudman Road, an unpaved one-lane track through a farm. Continue 1 mile to the trailhead on the right.

East of Orlando (Hikes 11-18)

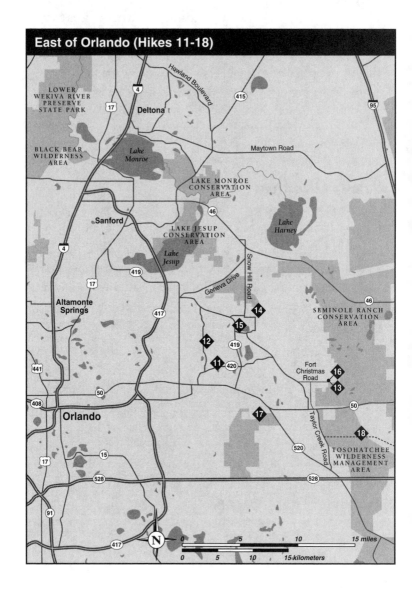

LOWER WEKIVA RIVER PRESERVE STATE PARK

Deltona

Howland Boulevard

BLACK BEAR WILDERNESS AREA

Lake Monroe

Maytown Road

LAKE MONROE CONSERVATION AREA

Sanford

LAKE JESUP CONSERVATION AREA

Lake Jesup

Lake Harney

Altamonte Springs

Geneva Drive

Snow Hill Road

SEMINOLE RANCH CONSERVATION AREA

Orlando

Fort Christmas Road

Taylor Creek Road

TOSOHATCHEE WILDERNESS MANAGEMENT AREA

N

0   5   10   15 miles

0   5   10   15 kilometers

East

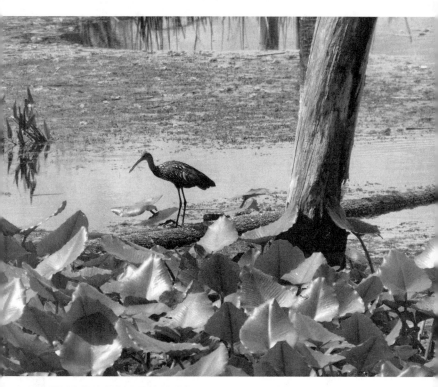

LIMPKIN AT ORLANDO WETLANDS PARK

Econlockhatchee
Sandhills
Conservation Area

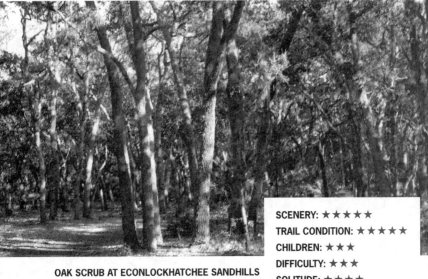

SCENERY: ★ ★ ★ ★ ★
TRAIL CONDITION: ★ ★ ★ ★ ★
CHILDREN: ★ ★
DIFFICULTY: ★ ★ ★
SOLITUDE: ★ ★ ★ ★

OAK SCRUB AT ECONLOCKHATCHEE SANDHILLS

GPS TRAILHEAD COORDINATES: N28° 35.258' W81° 09.353'

DISTANCE & CONFIGURATION: 3.2-mile balloon

HIKING TIME: 2 hours

HIGHLIGHTS: Oak scrub, open prairie, "wiggly trees"

ACCESS: Free; open daily, sunrise–sunset

MAPS: USGS *Oviedo*; sjrwmd.com/trailguides/pdfs/econlockhatchee_sandhillstrail.pdf

FACILITIES: None

WHEELCHAIR ACCESS: None

COMMENTS: Spectacular spot for fall wildflowers and fungi. Dogs not permitted.

CONTACTS: Orange County Environmental Protection Division, Green PLACE Program
(407) 836-1400

Overview

Nestled up against the floodplain of the Econlockhatchee River, the Econlockhatchee Sandhills Conservation Area is a 706-acre showcase of upland habitat diversity east of Orlando. Don't let the short access walk down a power line fool you: this is one of the prettiest day hikes in the region. The high, dry loop trail weaves through sand pine scrub, well-established oak hammocks, pine flatwoods, and pine savannas, while also providing glimpses of the grand cypresses outlining the nearby waterway.

Route Details

From the trailhead kiosk, which has detailed information and a map, the trail quickly jogs to the right beneath the tall longleaf pines. Cabbage palms are intermingled with the pines, and wiregrass, looking resplendent in fall, carpets the forest floor. A slight elevation change causes a transition into sand pine scrub. Sand live oaks cast shade on the footpath. In fall, blazing star and yellow aster lend bright splashes of color. Ignore the first unmarked trail junction amid the soft, fluffy sand pines, and veer right. The trail winds around and passes a small knoll covered in lichens before emerging under the power lines.

Cross beneath the power lines and veer left. Look for the red marker on the fence on the far side. Follow the sandy footpath through delicate, feathery grasses, including sprays of lovegrass. Prickly pear cactus grows on open, sandy spots. The next blaze is on the power line, and you must walk beneath it to cross a culvert at 0.5 mile. Watch for the red blaze to lead you back into the woods on the right before the next set of power poles. A double blaze leads you left off the forest road and onto a narrow footpath.

The footpath winds through the sandhills past older turkey oaks and tall longleaf pines. Just before you emerge into a patch of sun, you come to a double yellow marker. This marks the beginning of the loop portion of the hike, at 0.7 mile. Take the left fork. Yellow blazes lead you forward into a beautiful sand live oak hammock with

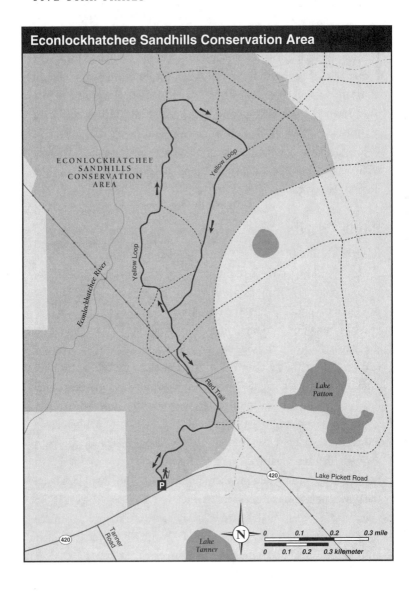

Econlockhatchee Sandhills Conservation Area

ECONLOCKHATCHEE
SANDHILLS
CONSERVATION
AREA

Yellow Loop

Yellow Loop

Econlockhatchee River

Red Trail

Lake
Patton

420 Lake Pickett Road

420

Tanner
Road

Lake
Tanner

N

0   0.1   0.2   0.3 mile

0   0.1   0.2   0.3 kilometer

an open understory. Crossing over an access road, continue straight. At a T-intersection with a path from the left, a double blaze points you to the right into a forest of young sand pine. The forest closes in around you, well shaded and canopied by sand live oaks, the ground covered in dense seafoam-colored puffs of deer moss. Look off to the left, and you'll see a line of trees getting taller and taller, a bayhead made up of loblolly bay with their white blooms. The trail reaches the bayhead at a wall of saw palmetto before turning to the right.

As the footpath becomes sandy underfoot, you notice the stillness all around, with only the chirp of crickets and warble of songbirds to rival the wind in the trees. Saw palmetto hems in from both sides. On the left, tall sweetgum trees outline the floodplain of the Econlockhatchee River. At 1.1 miles, the trail enters a stretch of full sun as it makes a sharp left to lead you into a pine savanna. A double blaze leads left, and it's here you see a forest of "wiggly trees," oaks growing so close together that their trunks resemble something out of a Dr. Seuss book. The habitat transitions to scrubby flatwoods, with the floodplain forest to your left. The tallest trees in the distance are cypresses, which grow along the banks of the river.

Inside the next oak hammock, it's a pure visual delight of shade and beauty. Hanging gardens of mosses cover the limbs of the older oaks, while the entire forest floor, as far as you can see, is puffy with deer moss. Turning sharply right at a marker, the trail leaves the hammock and heads out into the sandhills again, with oaks all around. Curving left, you're back into the wonderland of moss in the oak scrub. As the hammock opens up and becomes more parklike, you see the remnants of a deer stand on the left in a tree, and then you dive into the mossy hammock once again.

Turning left, the trail affords one last view of the cypresses before it curves right and away from the floodplain. The footpath goes from being crunchy with sand live oak leaves to grassy and mowed. Younger longleaf is establishing a foothold. This part of the hike is sun-drenched, the footpath tacking between patches of shade. As the trail swings left at a marker, an old road comes in from the right. Continue through the sandhills, with its large, open spaces filled with wildflowers, including flat-topped clusters of goldenrod. The trail follows an old road past stands of lopsided Indian grass and blazing stars.

At a four-way junction of forest roads, the double yellow blazes lead right. You see a confirmation blaze soon after. Turn right and follow this forest road past tall turkey oaks. The footpath is hard-packed, so it's easy walking. Around 2 miles, you pass a line of young longleaf pines on the right on the edge of a low scrub. A pine savanna continues on into the distance on the right. There are more "wiggly trees" on the left. At the fork in the road, keep left. The oaks crowd closely, forming a shady canopy.

After 2.4 miles, you reach the end of the loop. Turn left to exit. Be sure to turn right at the T-intersection to emerge under the power line. Head left under the power line and watch for the footpath on the far side of the culvert. Cross under the power line to follow the footpath back to the trailhead, completing the hike after 3.2 miles.

Nearby Attractions

The Econlockhatchee River is a popular destination for paddlers in the region. A longtime outfitter at Hidden River RV Park along FL 50 provides rentals and information about river conditions: (407) 568-5346. Download a map of the river from the Office of Greenways and Trails at **dep.state.fl.us/gwt/guide/designated_paddle/Econlock_guide.pdf.**

Directions

From the junction of FL 408 and FL 50, follow FL 50 east for 1.1 miles toward Titusville. Turn north on Lake Pickett Road (FL 420). Follow this road for 2.6 miles as it curves through a residential area before crossing the bridge over the Little Econlockhatchee River and entering a rural area. The ample trailhead parking area is on the left.

Econ River Wilderness Area

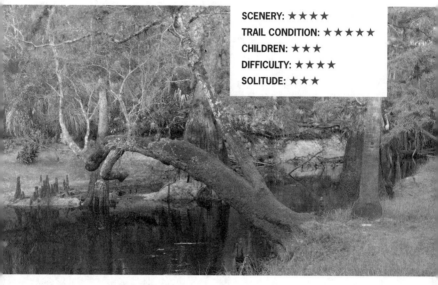

SCENERY: ★ ★ ★ ★
TRAIL CONDITION: ★ ★ ★ ★ ★
CHILDREN: ★ ★
DIFFICULTY: ★ ★ ★ ★
SOLITUDE: ★ ★ ★

LITTLE ECONLOCKHATCHEE RIVER

GPS TRAILHEAD COORDINATES: N28° 36.824' W81° 10.443'

DISTANCE & CONFIGURATION: 2.8-mile double loop (barbell)

HIKING TIME: 1.5 hours

HIGHLIGHTS: River views, ancient cypress, fall and summer wildflowers

ACCESS: Free; open daily, sunrise–sunset

MAPS: USGS *Oviedo SW*

FACILITIES: None

WHEELCHAIR ACCESS: None

COMMENTS: Portions of the trail may flood during the summer months.

CONTACTS: Seminole County Natural Lands Program (407) 349-0769;
seminolecountyfl.gov/parksrec/naturallands/econ.aspx

Econ River Wilderness Area

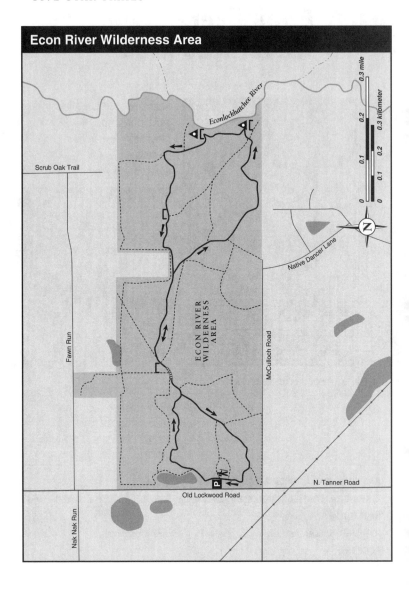

Overview

In the busy suburbs of Orlando, the Econ River Wilderness Area is an unlikely survivor. It protects 240 acres tucked one road back from strip malls and squeezed between subdivisions on the county line. A natural drainage area, it draws moisture downward through pine flatwoods toward the Econlockhatchee River. The well-maintained trail system leads you through a spectrum of habitats, with sweeping views across the pine flatwoods and quiet spots to rest along the river's banks.

Route Details

Start your hike by signing in at the trailhead kiosk, where the trail begins its lazy meander into a pine savanna. Passing a lily-dotted pond, the footpath turns right to head into the heart of this habitat, the high canopy made up of towering longleaf pine and the understory a dense sea of saw palmetto. By 0.25 mile, the trail slips into sandhills, where a cluster of sand live oaks provides a spot of shade amid the more colorful turkey oaks. You feel a constant drop in elevation as you walk.

Reaching the junction with the red-blazed trail at 0.4 mile, you will be at the bottom end of the top loop. Turn left to start walking down a forest road into a bayhead, one of Florida's swamp-forest habitats. At the four-way junction, take a right to follow a bridge over the drainage area onto a boardwalk through the bayhead swamp. Goldenrod and star rush peep out of the understory beneath dahoon holly in berry and the tall loblolly bay trees.

As you exit the boardwalk, turn right to continue, and keep right at the fork to follow the orange trail markers. The trail is nicely carpeted with a fine grass between the pines. In summer, pine lilies might surprise you with a flash of red. As the low spot, the trail can get mushy here after a rain. Passing an unmarked trail, you reach the top of the Flatwoods Loop. Keep to the right. Ignore the many side trails here and there, and stick with the main path. The understory beneath the pines is very dense with saw palmetto and gallberry. Past an enormous gopher tortoise burrow, you reach the "urban/wildland interface," where a large subdivision sits just beyond the property fence, which marks the county line between Seminole and Orange Counties. At the T-intersection along the fence, turn left.

Pulling away from the fence, the trail makes a left back into the pine woods, continuing on a steady, slow downhill to the river on the River Swamp Loop. You descend through another bayhead, where the roots of loblolly bay trees might trip you up as the trail closes in on the river. The trail opens up to a view of the river at 1.2 miles. The Econlockhatchee is a floodplain river, fed by rainfall, so water levels can vary wildly. When the water is low, you can see the ancient cypresses clearly. They are not very tall, but their bases are unusually broad and bulbous, perhaps stunted by the bedrock beneath the river bottom. A bench provides a perch for you to sit and savor this beauty spot until the mosquitoes chase you off.

Walk uphill through the cabbage palm hammock and take the right fork at the loop, walking through a river hammock with wax myrtle beneath the cabbage palms. Popping out of a thicket of saw palmetto, you have a nice view of the river again from atop a bluff. The habitat transitions to scrub, and you start passing side trails on the left. Keep heading straight, as there is one more beauty spot up ahead with a bench perched above the river and a heavily eroded slope below.

The uphill is noticeable, the trail as broad as a forest road as you pass a bat house. Sand live oaks grow in shortened clusters as though topped off by heavy winds. At a fork, follow the sweep of white sand left and uphill into a high, dry oak hammock with taller trees laden with Spanish moss, their limbs arching over the trail. As the elevation increases, you return to scrubby flatwoods with lots of blueberry bushes. You pass a bench under an oak tree at 1.9 miles. Reaching a T-intersection soon after, keep right.

Making a sharp left and right through the sandhills, the footpath emerges onto the main trail again, completing the lower loop.

Continue straight ahead, passing a reverse fork in the trail. An arrow points you left toward the boardwalk through the bayhead. Turn left off the boardwalk and bridge to continue uphill on the forest road. Pass the trail you came in on at 2.4 miles, and keep heading uphill. This is the one part of the preserve where the wildflowers are especially spectacular in fall: blazing star, Indian paintbrush, sabatia, and golden aster, along with very showy lopsided Indian grass (a tall grass that looks like a bird's feather). You see the caretaker's house off to the right as you ramble through the pine savanna, returning to the trailhead after 2.8 miles.

Nearby Attractions

This hike is right outside the campus of the University of Central Florida. A little-known free-to-the-public gem on campus is the UCF Arboretum, with more than 35 acres of botanical beauty among natural habitats: **arboretum.ucf.edu.**

Directions

From the intersection of FL 434 (Alafaya Trail) and FL 50 near the University of Central Florida, drive east on FL 434 and turn right on E. McCulloch Road. Drive 2 miles and turn left on Old Lockwood Road. The trailhead is on the right.

Florida Trail: Bronson State Forest

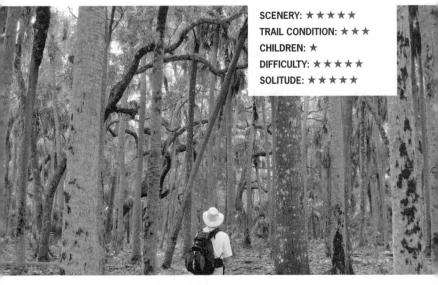

SCENERY: ★ ★ ★ ★ ★
TRAIL CONDITION: ★ ★ ★
CHILDREN: ★
DIFFICULTY: ★ ★ ★ ★ ★
SOLITUDE: ★ ★ ★ ★

AMONG THE ANCIENTS ON THE FLORIDA TRAIL

GPS TRAILHEAD COORDINATES:

Seminole Ranch Trailhead: N28° 34.142' W80° 59.791'

Joshua Creek Trailhead: N28° 35.5112' W81° 2.549'

Chuluota Wilderness Trailhead: N28° 37.393' W81° 03.797'

DISTANCE & CONFIGURATION: 13.7-mile one-way, with shuttle

HIKING TIME: 8.5 hours

HIGHLIGHTS: Palm hammocks, ancient live oaks, diverse wildflowers, Christmas Creek

ACCESS: $2 per person (only if accessed at midpoint); open 24/7

MAPS: USGS *Titusville SW, Aurantia,* and *Geneva*

FACILITIES: Picnic tables and campsites

WHEELCHAIR ACCESS: None

COMMENTS: The trail crosses rugged terrain prone to flooding; check water levels for the St. Johns River before setting out. This hike involves three land management areas with different regulations. Hunting is permitted in Seminole Ranch

Conservation Area and Charles H. Bronson State Forest; check hunt dates before hiking and use appropriate precautions. Free-range cattle roam most of the length of the trail. The length and difficulty of the hike call for an early start and a sensible pace so you finish before dark.

CONTACTS: Seminole Ranch Conservation Area, St. Johns River Water Management District (386) 329-4404 and **sjrwmd.com/recreationguide/seminoleranch;** Charles H. Bronson State Forest (407) 892-2963; Chuluota Wilderness Area (407) 349-0769 and **seminolecountyfl.gov/parksrec/naturallands/chuluota.aspx**

Overview

Dancing along the rim of the St. Johns River floodplain, the Florida Trail through Bronson State Forest—accessed via Seminole Ranch Conservation Area on the south end and Chuluota Wilderness Area on the north end—provides an unexpected array of botanical delights. Ancient oaks knit their limbs together to form grandly shaded hammocks. Towering cabbage palms rise like columns as far as the eye can see. The trail drops into leafy glades between creek drainages and climbs through spectacular stretches of pine savanna and diminutive scrub forests. This is one of Central Florida's most rugged and scenic day hikes.

Route Details

Since this is a linear trail, hiking the full 13.7-mile route requires leaving a car at the Chuluota Wilderness Trailhead. If you'd rather just hike 9.4 miles for the day, leave a car at the Joshua Creek Trailhead instead. See "Directions" on page 100.

Beginning at the trailhead at Seminole Ranch Conservation Area, follow the blue blaze from the kiosk in the corner of the parking area for an amble through cattle country. Crossing a cow pasture, you slip through deciduous forest between the cattle and Wheeler Road until the trail comes to a stile near an old cow pen. Climb over and continue into the forest on the other side. By 0.5 mile, you're walking in a wonderland of ancient oaks amid the palms, laden in resurrection fern and bromeliads. The earth gets darker underfoot. Crossing an old bridge over an ephemeral stream, the trail continues through

Florida Trail: Bronson State Forest

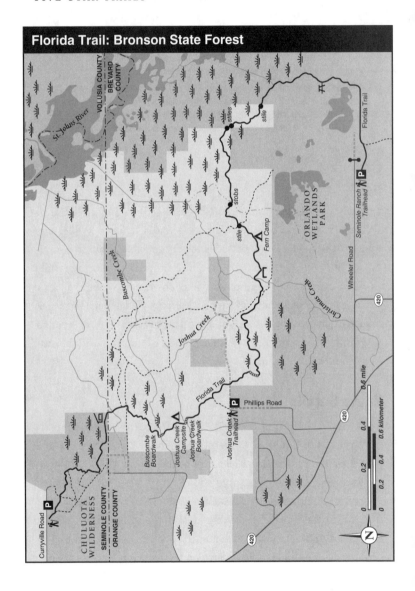

a very rooty area—watch your footing. At 0.9 mile you reach the junction with the main Florida Trail. Turn left to start hiking north through a series of palm hammocks, where you'll climb over the next stile before heading into a grove of ancient live oaks.

The trail emerges at a parking area adjoining the **Garden Spot Trail** at 1.7 miles, just beyond a cable gate. The orange blazes lead you onto a small bridge over a ditch filled with blue flag iris. Massive live oaks, cabbage palms, and cedars make up the forest. The open understory lets you peep out at pastureland and prairies along the St. Johns River. Pay attention so you don't smack into "the hugging tree," a big oak with limbs that try to embrace you. By 2.4 miles, you reach a picnic table between the trail and a forest road, which the trail begins to parallel. The next palm hammock resembles a natural cathedral, the towering trees blotting out the sky. Toothed rein orchid rises from the forest floor. Emerging onto the forest road, the trail uses the road to traverse a wetland before turning left into the woods and following the top of a low berm beneath the forest canopy. A footbridge and a trail sign mark the outflow of water from Orlando Wetlands Park. This is reclaimed wastewater, so don't fill your water bottles here. A side trail with blue blazes heads into the park. Continue following the orange blazes.

Cedars, cabbage palms, and oaks tower overhead as the trail continues through these hydric hammocks, so named for their tendency to be waterlogged much of the year. If the trail is even a few inches underwater, it will take much longer to complete it. Notice the water marks on the trees to see how deep it can get when the St. Johns River floods. The footing is rugged through most of the hydric hammocks, crossing many hummocks. You clamber over three stiles within the course of 15 minutes. Immediately after a stile, you reach the first intersection with the **River Trail**, a large loop within Bronson State Forest. Stay with the orange blazes to remain on the **Florida Trail**.

Entering a bower of enormous live oaks at 5.9 miles, the trail reaches Fern Camp, a primitive campsite. Rising out of the live oaks into open sky for the first time on the hike, you enter scrubby flatwoods dominated by tall pines. You see the first intrusion of the outside world since you entered this ribbon of green, a cell tower rising in the distance. Coming up to a long bench along a creek, you've found Christmas Creek at 6.5 miles, a good water source. Take a moment to sit and enjoy the scenery. It was along this creek that, during the First Seminole War in 1825, soldiers built a wooden stockade on Christmas Day.

Passing through another low-lying area with cypresses, the trail emerges into a pine savanna with delicate grasses poking between the mass of saw palmetto. Carnivorous plants find this habitat ideal. Watch for a pitcher plant bog in the low spots. More communications towers are visible in the distance. The trail turns northwest and comes up to a forest road crossing at an old gate. Watch for the trail sign and follow the footpath down the corridor along the fence line. As the trail gains elevation, the habitat transitions from scrubby flatwoods to pine savanna to sandhills in quick succession, with another drop through a small floodplain forest and a walk across a boardwalk at South Slough. By 9.2 miles, you reach a blue-blazed connector trail with the Joshua Creek Trailhead. This is a bailout point for a shorter day hike. It's an easy and well-marked 0.2-mile walk through the sandhills to the trailhead parking area.

Continue along the orange blazes as they lead you from the sandhills across more broad, open pine savanna. Pond pines rise from an impenetrable waist-deep sea of saw palmetto through which the trail cuts a swath. As the footpath loses elevation, you can see a ribbon of bayhead swamp on the horizon. In an open, overgrown pasture restoring itself to prairie, there is a profusion of wildflowers in every season. Prairie clover, blazing star, paw-paw, St. John's wort, and bog buttons rank among them. The trail drops down into the Joshua Creek floodplain, crossing this excellent water source on a series of two long boardwalks. At the end of the second boardwalk, a short blue-blazed trail leads west to the Joshua Creek Campsite.

Rising up into the shade of live oaks, the trail crosses the white-blazed equestrian loop and finds its way to the next floodplain.

Scrambling off the boardwalk across the marshes of Bunscombe Creek at 10.2 miles, you pass a particularly large and sprawling southern magnolia atop a small hill. A river of ferns cuts a green swath through the floodplain forest on your right, and the trail is mushy in places until it reaches the next hardwood hammock. Crossing the second intersection with the **River Trail** (marked in blue and white), the **Florida Trail** continues to a pass-through on the property line, emerging into Chuluota Wilderness Area at a covered bench at 11.3 miles.

Following an old forest road through a forest dominated by hickories and oaks, the trail keeps close to the property line, a barbed wire fence with the adjoining cattle ranch. As the footpath gains elevation, you enter the scrub, Florida's desert habitat. While tunneling beneath a canopy of diminutive oaks, notice their delicate hanging gardens of lichens and mosses. Descending through hickory and water oaks, southern magnolia, and a smattering of sweetgum trees, you can see a swampy bayhead off to the right as you walk through the shade and cross an equestrian trail, part of the loop trail system at Chuluota Wilderness.

The trail climbs into the heart of a healthy scrub forest atop ancient white sands. It's here you'll wind through one of Florida's rarest habitats, the rosemary scrub. These large, mounded bushes resemble sagebrush more than they do culinary rosemary, but they sport delicate blossoms. Deer moss thrives on this forest floor, its seafoam-colored bubbles popping up along and on the footpath. Between two firebreaks, the scrub forest is regenerating. Older sand pines tower over the Florida rosemary as the trail winds its way upward across the ancient dunes, crossing one more forest road before it emerges at the Chuluota Wilderness Area trailhead kiosk, wrapping up this 13.7-mile hike.

Nearby Attractions

Fort Christmas Historical Park (**nbbd.com/godo/FortChristmas**) is a popular stop during the holiday season for an immersion into pioneer history and the opportunity to play inside a replica of the fort built on Christmas Creek. The park is open daily at 8 a.m. and includes restroom, picnic, and playground facilities. The historic structures are closed on Mondays and holidays, as is the gift shop. Two other entries in this book, Orlando Wetlands Park (Hike 16, page 111) and Florida Trail: Mills Creek Woodlands (Hike 14, page 101) are located near the endpoints of this hike.

Directions

To Seminole Ranch Trailhead (south end): From the intersection of FL 50 and Fort Christmas Road in Christmas, follow Fort Christmas Road north for 2.3 miles. Pass Fort Christmas Park on the left and turn right, along the curve, at the sign for Orlando Wetlands Park. Follow Wheeler Road for 1.5 miles to the parking area for Seminole Ranch Conservation Area, across the road from the entrance to Orlando Wetlands Park.

To Joshua Creek Trailhead (midpoint): From Seminole Ranch Trailhead, turn left. Drive 3.1 miles west to Phillips Road. Turn right. Continue 1.5 miles along Phillips Road to the sign for Bronson State Forest. Take the jeep track to the left of the sign. It empties into a very large parking area with a couple of picnic tables. Be sure to pay the day-use fee and sign the register before you leave a car here.

To Chuluota Wilderness Trailhead (north end): From the turn-off for Phillips Road on Fort Christmas Road, continue 5.8 miles to Lake Mills Road. Turn right and drive 0.8 mile to Curryville Road. Turn right and continue 2.5 miles to the trailhead entrance for Chuluota Wilderness Area on the right.

14

Florida Trail: Mills Creek Woodlands

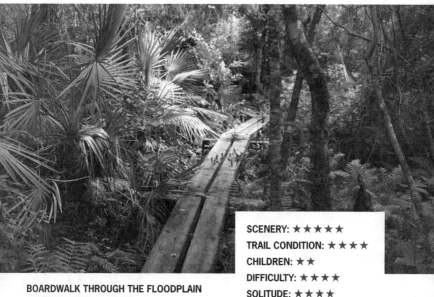

SCENERY: ★ ★ ★ ★ ★
TRAIL CONDITION: ★ ★ ★ ★
CHILDREN: ★ ★
DIFFICULTY: ★ ★ ★ ★
SOLITUDE: ★ ★ ★ ★

BOARDWALK THROUGH THE FLOODPLAIN FOREST OF MILLS CREEK

GPS TRAILHEAD COORDINATES: N28° 39.186' W81° 05.804'

DISTANCE & CONFIGURATION: 4-mile out-and-back

HIKING TIME: 3 hours

HIGHLIGHTS: Boardwalks through swamp forests, Mills Creek

ACCESS: Free; open 24/7

MAPS: USGS *Geneva*

FACILITIES: Picnic table and primitive campsite with benches

WHEELCHAIR ACCESS: None

COMMENTS: Parking is very limited unless you use the central trailhead, which involves a difficult mile-long out-and-back walk through rough pastureland. The boardwalks along this trail can be slippery and time-consuming to cross.

CONTACTS: USDA Forest Service, National Forests in Florida (850) 523-8500 and **fs.usda .gov/fnst**; Florida Trail Association (877) HIKE-FLA and **floridatrail.org**

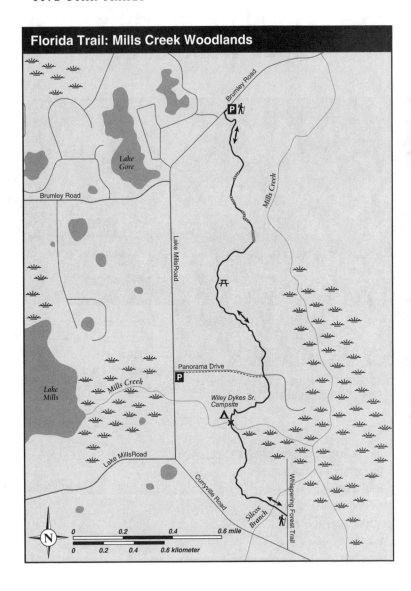

Florida Trail: Mills Creek Woodlands

Overview

As the Florida Trail follows the curve of the basin into which Mills Creek drains from Lake Mills, it leads you through a colorful array of habitats. There are oak hammocks where ancient oaks seem to bend under the weight of streamers of Spanish moss, bayhead swamps with ferns growing in massive tufts, diminutive desertlike scrub where prickly pear cactus and tarflower thrive, and lush hardwoods providing deep shade. Although this segment of the Florida Trail is only 2 miles long, it's a tricky one to negotiate and is so packed with diversity you'll find yourself spending hours engaged with its beauty.

Route Details

From Brumley Road, follow the orange blazes of the **Florida Trail** south, away from the pasture and into the woods through a pass-through in the fence. Heading downhill fast—uncommon on Florida's trails—your surroundings abruptly shift from sandhills to a hardwood hammock. The trail comes to a T with a broader path. Turn right and follow the orange blazes. You're in a tunnel in deep shade beneath arching oak branches laden with resurrection fern. Curving left beneath showy live oaks, the trail continues to lose elevation as habitats collide along the ecotone. Keep right at the fork. Tall live oaks draped in Spanish moss provide shade and a virtual hanging garden of ferns, bromeliads, and orchids, a beauty spot along the walk.

The trail makes a sharp left off the wide path and becomes a narrow path winding through saw palmetto and ferns, with rugged footing due to the trunks of the saw palmetto and many roots in the footpath. Jogging around a significant-sized oak tree, you're still losing elevation as you walk. Soon after, the first boardwalk begins. These are not your average boardwalks. Built by F-Troop, the Florida Trail Association volunteer trail crew, they are nicely elevated over the rough, mushy terrain of the bayhead swamp but require a good sense of balance and attention to footing. The first boardwalk is made of two sturdy but narrow planks with a gap between. Consider it a two-footed balance beam. And it is slippery. Traverse carefully, using your hiking stick, so you don't slide off into the swamp. By no means a straight line, the boardwalk zigs around stands of loblolly bay and zags around big sprays of ferns reaching shoulder height. Songbirds sing from the dark depths of the bayhead. It is always dark, cool, and a bit buggy but still a magical place to immerse yourself in—a natural fernery of timeless beauty.

The first boardwalk ends and drops you into an island of pines before you start the next boardwalk, which is slick from humidity and moss. Even in times of drought, pools of standing water collect here and nourish aquatic plants. After 0.5 mile, the boardwalk ends at a stand of very old and tall pines. Turn right at the T-intersection and head down a straightaway, following the blazes. Swamp azalea flourishes in a spot along this section on the right, blooming in summer and attracting a steady parade of butterflies.

As you ascend a hill through a forest with an open understory, you can see pasture off to the right at the top of the hill, a reminder that you're not as deep in the woods as you might have thought. Passing an old barbed wire fence, the trail jogs to the left before emerging into the grassy pasture. Rather than ascend the top of the knoll, the trail keeps to the left. As you arrive at a picnic table, stop a moment and watch for deer coming over the rise. Beyond the picnic table, the trail continues through young hardwood forest. The hill drops sharply off to the left into the creek basin. After 1 mile, pass through a gateway created out of a bit of fence. Crossing a narrow sand road, you come up to the intersection with the blue-blazed side trail at 1.2 miles from the main parking area.

Continuing down an old road, the trail comes to a bayhead and enters it, soggy underfoot. A small plank bridge crosses the outflow; beyond it, the footpath is full of ankle-turning roots as it makes a sharp left into a younger forest. The understory is open, so watch for the orange blazes. After passing under southern magnolias, you reach the Wiley Dykes Sr. Campsite at 1.4 miles. A short blue blaze leads you to the site, which has benches and a fire ring. Beyond the campsite, the trail quickly works its way to the floodplain of Mills Creek, which flows out of Lake Mills and creates a large basin swamp. You'll know you're in the floodplain when cypress knees start poking out of the footpath. It's a beautiful place, filled with ferns and tall cypresses. Beware of the poison ivy that grows thickly here—and watch your footing. The slippery bridge has leveled a few hikers. Though the addition of hardware cloth has made it safer, it's nonetheless worthy of respect for a small bridge.

Leaving the floodplain, the trail climbs up and up, beneath massive southern magnolia and hickory trees. You can smell the change in the air as the trail gains more elevation and enters a scrub, Florida's desert. Tufts of deer moss appear across the blinding white sand. Diminutive oaks and fluffy sand pines offer no shade. Tunneling through the sand pine forest, you emerge at the end of this Florida Trail segment at Whispering Pines Trail, a private drive, at 2 miles. This is your turnaround point. Backtracking through the scrub forest, the floodplain of Mills Creek, the gentle pastureland, and the slippery boardwalks through the heart of the swamp, you return to your car after a tricky but spectacular 4-mile hike.

Nearby Attractions

Two other entries in this book are nearby: Lake Mills Park (Hike 15, page 106) and Florida Trail: Bronson State Forest (Hike 13, page 94).

Directions

From downtown Oviedo, head east on County Road 419 for 6.2 miles, passing through Chuluota. Turn left onto Lake Mills Road and drive 1.8 miles. Follow the curve of the road to the left. Continue 1.2 miles, passing a trailhead for this Florida Trail section on the right. The road becomes Brumley Road. Follow it another 0.4 mile, around the curve under the oaks, and park on the left at the trail crossing, off the road.

Lake Mills Park

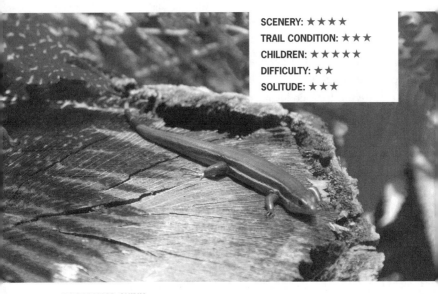

SCENERY: ★ ★ ★
TRAIL CONDITION: ★ ★ ★
CHILDREN: ★ ★ ★ ★ ★
DIFFICULTY: ★ ★
SOLITUDE: ★ ★ ★

BROADHEAD SKINK

GPS TRAILHEAD COORDINATES: N28° 37.986' W81° 07.386'

DISTANCE & CONFIGURATION: 0.8-mile loop and spur

HIKING TIME: 45 minutes

HIGHLIGHTS: Gentle boardwalks through cypress swamp, observation deck on Lake Mills

ACCESS: Free; open 8 a.m.–sunset; closed Thanksgiving and December 25

MAPS: USGS *Geneva*

FACILITIES: Campground, picnic pavilions, playground, restrooms

WHEELCHAIR ACCESS: Boardwalks are wheelchair-accessible. Best approach is via campground.

COMMENTS: Beautiful campground for tent camping and small campers ($15 per night, includes bathhouse with hot showers). Pets and alcohol are not permitted. The lake is not open for swimming.

CONTACTS: Lake Mills Park (407) 665-2001; **seminolecountyfl.gov/parksrec/ PassiveParksandBoatRamps/lakemillspark.aspx**

Overview

One of Seminole County's prettiest county parks, Lake Mills Park perches along the southwest shore of Lake Mills, where a hardwood swamp dominated by tall cypresses provides a focal point for a series of boardwalks that showcase its beauty. Snuggled into the saw palmetto and oaks, the campground is especially inviting, and the park is always busy with families enjoying the modern playground, big picnic pavilions, and lakefront on which to fish or launch a kayak.

Route Details

As you leave the parking area, you're surrounded by the elements of a county park: picnic tables, restrooms, and a large fenced-in playground with a climbing wall and bouncy dinosaur. You will find lots of fun for the kids, with equipment for both toddlers and older children.

Take a left past the playground to walk down to the lake. Glimpse its shimmering waters beyond the grand live oaks shading the picnic area, oaks more than 150 years old. Crossing over the fitness trail that works its way through the park, continue down the slight incline to see the lake. Reaching a boardwalk, follow it out to the observation deck, which overlooks a cove along Lake Mills. It's a sweeping view, where buttonbushes dangle over the water's edge, the ivory-yellow blooms of American lotus slowly undulate on the gentle waves of the lake, and snowy egrets pick through the shallows. At the bases of the tall cypresses, just beyond the water line, royal ferns grow in profusion.

Leaving this beauty spot, make a left. There are two trees straight ahead of you, a cypress and an oak, tangled up in each other's embrace. You immediately come up to the first boardwalk. Turn right. Signs warn you that the boardwalk can be slippery when wet. Adjoining the boardwalk is a creek that flows into Lake Mills, with clear, slightly tannic water and a sand bottom. Mounds of royal ferns cluster along its shores, along with copious amounts of poison ivy, which climbs up the towering cypress, mimicking the leaves of the hickory trees. Being on the boardwalk keeps you out of harm's way.

Lake Mills Park

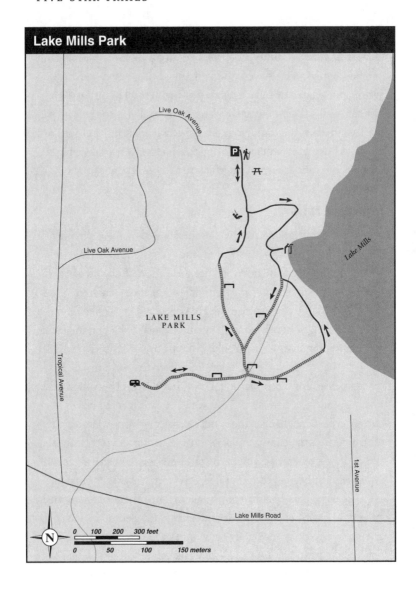

Live Oak Avenue

Live Oak Avenue

Lake Mills

LAKE MILLS
PARK

Tropical Avenue

1st Avenue

Lake Mills Road

0	100	200	300 feet

0	50	100	150 meters

N

There are many benches and observation platforms along the boardwalk. You reach the first at 0.25 mile, where you can marvel at the height of the cypresses overhead. At the T-intersection, make a left. An observation platform sits over the creek at this point. It's an appealing place to sit and watch leaves drift past while lizards and skinks scurry over the fallen logs. At the next T-intersection, turn right to follow the creek upstream. Sunlight dapples through the deep shade of the canopy above. Ferns flourish in this damp environment, filling the understory with a diverse mixture of species. A large deck beneath a massive cypress provides another overlook onto the creek.

Passing the next bench, you cross over the creek. A slight bit of movement belies the location of a leopard frog. To the left, a tree arches over the creek as it flows out of a dense thicket of bayhead swamp, the waterway lit by a patch of sun where turtles stretch out for warmth on a sandbar. During the summer, your senses will be drawn to a nice patch of swamp honeysuckle, the only member of the rhododendron family in Florida that blooms during the summer. Take a whiff, and you will see why it attracts colorful tiger swallowtail butterflies.

With the honeysuckle a backdrop to the transition, the boardwalk rises out of the swamp and into a scrub forest before emptying out into the campground next to Campsite 9 after 0.4 mile. This is the best access point for wheelchairs. Turn around and retrace your steps back downhill along the boardwalk, crossing over the creek again and passing the deck. At the T-intersection, turn right.

This is an older section of boardwalk with a bit of a cant to it, enabling you to see remnants of the old boardwalk under the new on the right as you come up to its first observation deck with a bench. Here, away from the creek, the water flow is sluggish, swampy beneath the dense forest canopy. The boardwalk swoops around several bends, facing an open space ahead as you draw closer to the lake. Past a towering cypress on the right, the mounds of royal fern are especially showy.

The boardwalk emerges at the edge of the lake, with the park boundary marked by a fence on the right. Turn left and enjoy the view as you walk down what was one of the original roads in the area, which you can tell when you cross the old concrete bridge over the creek. Citrus trees flank the waterway. There is an excellent view of the lake where the creek enters it, a spot favored by wading birds as they watch for fish darting from the outflow.

By 0.6 mile, you've completed the loop back to the original boardwalk you started on. For a slightly different perspective on the swamp, turn left and walk back upstream along that boardwalk. At the T-intersection, turn right. From this boardwalk, you can better see the line of big cypresses that you've been walking through. Clusters of ferns grow high off the swamp floor, showing how deep the water can get. The boardwalk ends along the edge of an outdoor classroom. When you come to a T-intersection and see the playground in front of you, turn right. Make the immediate left to walk back to your car, completing the easy 0.8-mile walk.

Nearby Attractions

Two other entries in this book are nearby: Florida Trail: Mills Creek Woodlands (Hike 14, page 101) and Florida Trail: Bronson State Forest (Hike 13, page 94). The Cross Seminole Trail, an excellent expedition for cyclists, passes right by the park entrance and heads toward the Snow Hill Road Trailhead for Little Big Econ State Forest.

Directions

From downtown Oviedo, head east on County Road 419 for 6.2 miles, passing through Chuluota. Turn left onto Lake Mills Road and drive 0.3 mile to Tropical Avenue. Turn left. The park entrance is on the right. Follow the park road around to the left, in the opposite direction from the campground, until you get to the last large pavilion that sits off by itself with a long strip of parking along the park road. For wheelchair access to the boardwalk, turn right, into the campground, and follow the road around to Campsite 9, where the boardwalk comes into the campground from the right.

Orlando Wetlands Park

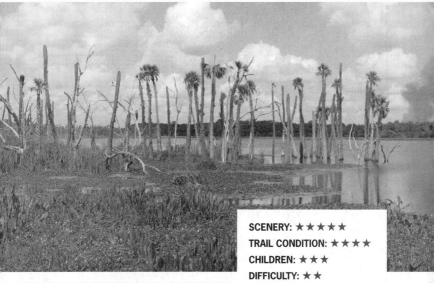

SCENERY: ★ ★ ★ ★ ★
TRAIL CONDITION: ★ ★ ★ ★
CHILDREN: ★ ★ ★
DIFFICULTY: ★ ★
SOLITUDE: ★ ★ ★ ★

SHALLOW MARSHES AT ORLANDO WETLANDS PARK

GPS TRAILHEAD COORDINATES: N28° 34.191' W80° 59.785'

DISTANCE & CONFIGURATION: 4.8-mile loop

HIKING TIME: 2.5 hours

HIGHLIGHTS: Excellent birding and expansive views

ACCESS: Free; open daily, sunrise–sunset; closed November 15–January 31

MAPS: USGS *Titusville SW*

FACILITIES: Restrooms and picnic pavilion

WHEELCHAIR ACCESS: None

COMMENTS: No pets allowed. Bicycles welcome.

CONTACTS: City of Orlando (407) 568-1706; **cityoforlando.net/public_works/wetlands**

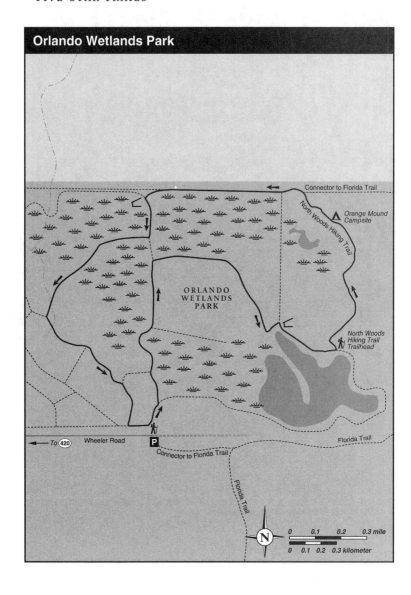

Orlando Wetlands Park

Connector to Florida Trail

North Woods Hiking Trail

Orange Mound
Campsite

ORLANDO
WETLANDS
PARK

North Woods
Hiking Trail
Trailhead

To 420   Wheeler Road

Florida Trail

Connector to Florida Trail

Florida Trail

N

0   0.1   0.2   0.3 mile

0   0.1   0.2   0.3 kilometer

Overview

The granddaddy of wetlands parks, Orlando Wetlands Park is a City of Orlando wastewater reclamation project that's become a world-class haven for waterfowl. The project began in the mid-1980s with the acquisition of a dairy farm. Converted to a series of wetland "cells" of varying depths, historic cattle ranches became marsh in which treated wastewater would filter naturally through native aquatic plants before being returned to the St. Johns River watershed. Covering more than 1,600 acres, the complex offers hiking on the dikes between the impoundments and in surrounding forests. This route provides a sampler of both, but there are many different approaches to exploring this park.

Route Details

For a hike filled with the flutter, squawk, and flash of birds busy about their daily routines, Orlando Wetlands Park is one of the best spots in the state. Starting off from the parking area, walk up to the pavilion and kiosk area near the restrooms. You'll find trail maps here, as well as information about the birds that frequent the park. Pass the restrooms and a picnic shelter, and you're on the Birding Trail Loop, which immediately comes to a Y intersection. Turn left.

As you come up to a bench, note the map outlining all of the possible routes in the park. You'll find many of these maps throughout the trail system, a genuine help to keep you on the right route. To your left, the impoundment has open water in the foreground and aquatic plants in the background, a place where mergansers, teals, ducks, and geese tend to gather. The open wetlands provide vast panoramas, edged with planted cabbage palms in the distance.

After 0.25 mile, you reach a T-intersection with another dike. Keep right to loop around the large, open wetland on the left. The wetland pool on the right is deeply covered in vegetation so you can't see across it. Past the next bench on the right is a cattail marsh with incursions of wax myrtle and palm hammock islands. The next bench overlooks a pond, where you might glimpse an alligator going after its breakfast. Look for the footprints of raccoons and the tracks of deer in the soft sand along the water's edge.

Skip the next two paths on the right. Continue past another bench and enjoy the views across the impoundment on the left, watching for Louisiana herons near shore and coots skittering between patches of pickerelweed. See the pines in the far distance? They mark the perimeter of the park. Turn right at the next dike, at 0.8 mile. At the next junction of dikes, watch for sandhill cranes browsing atop these taller dikes. Cattle egrets fly past with bits of reeds in their beaks to build nests on an island of cabbage palms off to your left, where they have a nesting colony. The pickerelweed grows in beautiful clusters throughout this area, adjacent to the dike. Straight ahead, you can see a patch of tall pines, so you know you're drawing close to the northern edge of the park.

The trail comes up to a large mound along the edge of an impoundment. There is a cypress dome well off in the distance as the trail comes up to a major intersection at 1.5 miles. Turn left. After you cross the culvert, turn right to head toward a rain shelter. This vast body of open water is Lake Searcy, and the dike trail follows it to meet the **North Woods Hiking Trail.** Turn left to start down this foot-path, meandering through hammocks of oaks and palms in a boggy, soggy meld of habitats where mosquitoes can be quite fierce. Bog bridges get you across the wettest spots.

By 2.1 miles, you're walking along a beautiful palm hammock with an ephemeral waterway on your left. Star rush and lilies peep up from the forest floor. The trail hops up onto a levee covered in oak trees. There's a double blaze where the trail crosses a small balance beam–style bridge (watch your footing) into a palm hammock on the other side. At 2.5 miles you reach the Orange Mound Campsite, a quiet primitive site for hikers slipping off the nearby Florida Trail. The trail enters a cathedral of cabbage palms, a very dense palm hammock.

Emerging from the palms, you reach a bridge over a small canal. Cross the bridge to meet a trail at a fence line. Turn left to continue creating a large loop, walking west with the fence line to your right and the stream to your left and plenty of shade overhead. At the next bridge, turn left at a sluiceway and start down this dike. After 3.3 miles, you reach a rain shelter at the upper end of the **Birding Trail Loop.** As you come up to the shelter, turn left, heading down that levee to pass a bench on the right-hand side. At the next levee, you rejoin the Birding Trail Loop. Turn right to head into the middle of the marshes. Near the outflow at 3.7 miles, a bench faces off into the cattail marsh, which is busy with moorhens.

At 4.1 miles, you reach a T-intersection with the next dike. Turn left for the return loop of the Birding Trail Loop. At 4.3 miles, the hammock on the left ends and the wetlands open up again; on the right, a dike leads off into the distance for exploration of the farther reaches of the park. Pass by it and stay on the path you're following. You cross another outflow culvert, busy with activity. Coming to a T-intersection, turn right and walk along the dike, with the cattail marsh to your right and a willow marsh to your left, toward the exit. At the next T-intersection, you face a wall of marsh vegetation. Turn left to leave the complex, emerging behind the restrooms and pavilion. Continue through to the parking area, wrapping up a 4.8-mile hike.

Nearby Attractions

Fort Christmas Historical Park (**nbbd.com/godo/FortChristmas**) is a popular stop during the holiday season for an immersion into pioneer history and for the opportunity to play inside a replica of the fort built on Christmas Creek. The park opens daily at 8 a.m. and has restroom, picnic, and playground facilities. The historical structures, however, are closed on Mondays and holidays, as is the gift shop. The entry on the Florida Trail: Bronson State Forest (Hike 13, page 94), the southern end of the Florida Trail, starts across the street from Orlando Wetlands Park.

Directions

From FL 408, follow FL 50 east toward Titusville for 11 miles. At Christmas, turn left on Fort Christmas Road (watch for the Christmas trees on the corner). Continue 2.3 miles, passing Fort Christmas Historical Park, to the turnoff straight ahead where the road otherwise makes a sharp left curve. Turn right on Wheeler Road and continue 1.7 miles down to the trailhead parking area on your left.

Pine Lily Preserve

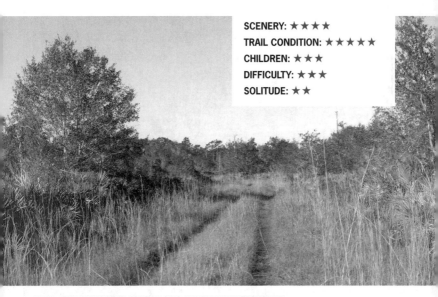

SCENERY: ★ ★ ★ ★
TRAIL CONDITION: ★ ★ ★ ★ ★
CHILDREN: ★ ★ ★
DIFFICULTY: ★ ★ ★
SOLITUDE: ★ ★

TRAIL THROUGH PINE FLATWOODS AT PINE LILY PRESERVE

GPS TRAILHEAD COORDINATES: N28° 31.717' W81° 05.772'

DISTANCE & CONFIGURATION: 4.3 miles in a balloon and an out-and-back

HIKING TIME: 2 hours

HIGHLIGHTS: Colorful wildflowers, carnivorous plants, historic road

ACCESS: Free; open daily, sunrise–sunset

MAPS: USGS *Bithlo*

FACILITIES: None

WHEELCHAIR ACCESS: None

COMMENTS: Dogs and bicycles are not permitted.

CONTACTS: Orange County Environmental Protection Division, Green PLACE Program
(407) 836-1400

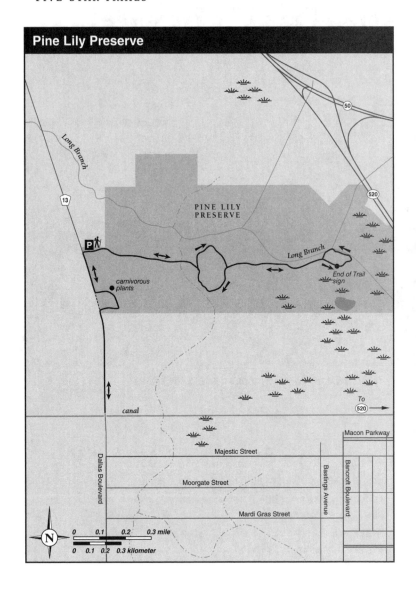

Pine Lily Preserve

Long Branch

50

13

520

PINE LILY
PRESERVE

Long Branch

P

carnivorous
plants

End of Trail
sign

To
520

canal

Macon Parkway

Majestic Street

Dallas Boulevard

Bastings Avenue

Bancroft Boulevard

Moorgate Street

Mardi Gras Street

N

| 0 | 0.1 | | 0.2 | 0.3 mile |

| 0 | 0.1 | 0.2 | 0.3 kilometer |

Overview

A showcase for the colorful pine lily (*Lilium catesbaei* Walter), a threatened species that thrives in wet flatwoods, Pine Lily Preserve protects 409 acres in the Econlockhatchee River basin. Connecting directly to Hal Scott Preserve and Long Branch Preserve, it is part of a much larger corridor for wildlife to roam north from the prairies of Osceola County. The pine lilies bloom in late summer, but there are always colorful wildflowers to be found in this preserve, particularly around the marshes and wet prairies.

Route Details

From the trailhead kiosk, where you'll find a map of the preserve and details about its inhabitants, walk toward and around the gate at the end of the parking area to a forest road surrounded by scattered saw palmettos and prairie grasses. Longleaf pine towers overhead, and you can hear the hum of FL 50 not far away. The trail markers, on posts, are discs, and they are not entirely consistent in color along the trails. So keep alert. It's not hard to follow this trail, however, as it's broad and pleasant. The tawny grasses flanking the trail cup small spiderwebs filled with morning dew.

The habitat transitions into pine flatwoods, tall slash pines that, by their spacing, might have been planted here decades ago. At 0.25 mile, the trail indents slightly into the woods on the left. The forest crowds close on the left but sweeps south into pine savanna on the right. As it loses elevation, the trail enters a floodplain with cabbage palms and cypresses overhead. Gravel is laid across the trail to enable the flow of a stream to seep through. Live oaks, their limbs laden with resurrection fern, knit a canopy above the trail as it gains elevation again.

After 0.5 mile, you reach the junction with the north half of the central loop in the trail, a trail marked with blue arrows. Turn left. This is a footpath in the woods, a wilder place. The footpath is a little rough, the trail paralleled by floodplain trees. The trail curves to the right, a slow turn to face east. A pine savanna now sweeps off to the left. Emerging at the main trail again, turn left on the broad path. Traffic noise increases as you draw close to FL 520, one of the busier highways in the region. The slight dampness of the soil encourages plants you'll find around pine lilies, including wild bachelor's button and St. John's wort, to bloom. At an unmarked junction with a cross trail, continue straight ahead. Rising up again, the trail reaches a fork at 1.2 miles.

Take the left fork, following the markers to amble to a berm along a creek. The trail turns right to follow the creek, a few cypresses outlining the floodplain. Keep watching for the next trail marker. The trail pulls away from paralleling the creek. Look for another marker, under a pine tree, guiding you toward a stand of young pines. You reach an END OF TRAIL sign off to your left at 1.4 miles, and complete this small loop at 1.5 miles.

As you return along the broad path, it doesn't take long to be immersed in grassy, open scrubby flatwoods with prairie grasses. Passing the north trail again, continue a little ways forward to find the south loop starting on the left. Turn left to head down between walls of shoulder-height saw palmetto with tall longleaf pines above, the panorama stretching off to the left until the oaks crowd in and form a canopy. The trail drops down slightly, dark earth making up the footpath, a little mucky on the shoes. Push past palm fronds and mossy banks where colorful fungi grow, and when you emerge at the main trail, turn left.

A small sweep of pine savanna is off to the left as you walk in the open sun, slender flat-topped goldenrod lending splashes of yellow in the foreground. Crossing over the gravel wash, you rise up into a corridor of oaks and reach the gate at the trailhead after 2.7 miles.

You could stop here, but you'd be missing out. The red trail heads south from this trailhead too. Follow the southern fence line toward the road until you find it, and follow the red markers down the power line for almost 0.25 mile. There, a cypress dome blocks southerly progress. A post with a marker points you into a sharp left to cross a marshy drainage area. It's here, in this drainage that flows out of the cypresses and into the prairie, that you'll find some of the nicest wildflowers in the preserve: the lilac-tinged blooms of lobelia, delicate yellow bladderworts, and the sticky crimson arms of carnivorous sundews among them.

Reaching a T-intersection with a closed trail, turn right for a walk through scrubby flatwoods, a potentially soggy habitat with high potential for pine lilies. By 3 miles, you reach the next T-intersection; red trail markers point right, toward the power line. This time, however, you continue under the power line and summit the roadbed of old County Road 13. Turn left. Whether the roadbed was built in the 1920s or 1940s, or was a railroad bed from even earlier days, it stands up tall around the surrounding landscape, which means expansive views for you as you walk down it. And an easy walk it is. Red diamond markers lead you down the nicely shaded corridor. At 3.3 miles, a panorama of palmetto prairie and wiregrass stretches off to the horizon on the right. As the canopy of oaks closes in again, the old roadbed bisects a cypress dome, the interplay of light and shadow most delicate through the feathery cypress needles.

A jarring contrast happens at 3.5 miles, when the trail reaches a vast swath of cleared land with a canal running perpendicular to the trail. It seems out of place. This is your turnaround point. It's an easy and straight walk back through the cypress dome and up to the south end of CR 13, visible just through the trees. Turn right to head down the hill, and left at the next intersection. Within a tenth of a mile, make a left at the post with the markers to walk back through the scrubby flatwoods, following the trail back through the wildflower wetland and up along the power line. You emerge at the trailhead parking area after 4.3 miles.

Nearby Attractions

One of the crazier evenings in the greater Orlando area can be had right around the corner at Orlando Speed World Dragway watching funny cars, dragsters, and even school bus demolition derbies as the lights come up after dark: **speedworlddragway.com.**

Directions

Follow FL 50 from Orlando or Titusville to Bithlo, west of FL 520. Turn south on CR 13. As you drive down it, it narrows to a small canopied road. You'll pass Long Branch Preserve on the right before finding Pine Lily Preserve on the left as the road ends. Be especially careful pulling into the parking area, as the pavement drops off steeply: Take it at an angle.

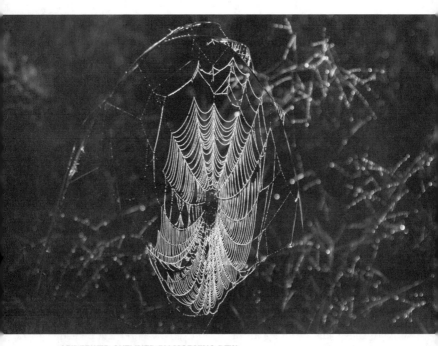

SPIDERWEB OUTLINED BY MORNING DEW

18 # Tosohatchee Wildlife Management Area

SCENERY: ★★★★★
TRAIL CONDITION: ★★★
CHILDREN: ★
DIFFICULTY: ★★★★★
SOLITUDE: ★★★★★

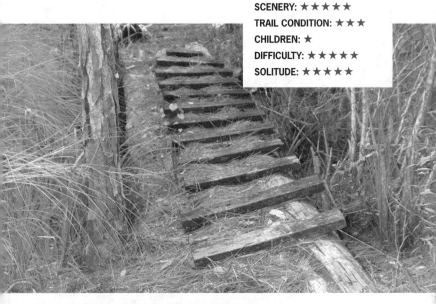

ONE OF THE OLDER BRIDGES AT TOSOHATCHEE WMA

GPS TRAILHEAD COORDINATES: N28° 30.237' W80° 57.008'

DISTANCE & CONFIGURATION: 11.7-mile loop

HIKING TIME: 8 hours

HIGHLIGHTS: Palm hammocks, ancient pine forests, solitude

ACCESS: $3 per person; open 24/7

MAPS: USGS *Titusville SW* and *Lake Poinsett NW*

FACILITIES: Restroom at entrance

WHEELCHAIR ACCESS: None

COMMENTS: This is a rugged wilderness area. Carry a map and compass or GPS. If the St. Johns River is flooded, it may not be possible to complete the full loop in a day. Poison ivy is common here. Wear long pants to protect your skin.

CONTACTS: Florida Fish and Wildlife Conservation Commission Regional Office (352) 732-1225; **myfwc.com/viewing/recreation/wmas/lead/Tosohatchee**

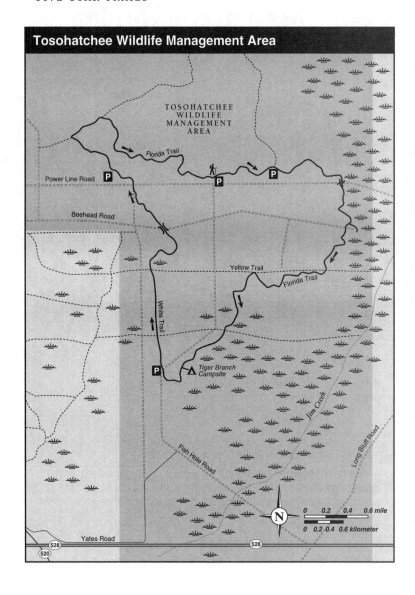

Tosohatchee Wildlife Management Area

TOSOHATCHEE
WILDLIFE
MANAGEMENT
AREA

Florida Trail

Power Line Road

Beehead Road

Yellow Trail

Florida Trail

White Trail

Tiger Branch
Campsite

Fish Hole Road

Jim Creek

Long Bluff Road

0   0.2   0.4   0.6 mile
0 0.2 0.4 0.6 kilometer

Yates Road

Overview

Protecting more than 30,000 acres of wild space along the St. Johns River between Orlando and Titusville, Tosohatchee Wildlife Management Area (WMA) is a grand expanse for hikers to play in. The Florida Trail runs through the preserve, as it has for many decades, beneath bowers of ancient live oaks, through mazes of cabbage palms, and among towering stands of slash pine. The creeks and streams are lined with old-growth cypress, including virgin cypress along Jim Creek. To enjoy a full day in Tosohatchee, a rugged place to hike, the White Loop provides almost 12 miles to explore, utilizing the Florida Trail as the eastern portion of the loop.

Route Details

From the parking area under the power line, a short blue-blazed trail slips northeast to connect you with the Florida Trail. Just a few footsteps and you are enveloped in the first of many spectacular palm hammocks for which Tosohatchee is known. Make a right here and start following the orange blazes, noting copious amounts of poison ivy on both sides of the trail and overhead in the trees. This is a trail with a true wilderness feel. The deeper into the preserve you go, the quieter it gets. The footpath is often just wide enough for your feet.

At 0.8 mile, a blue-blazed trail leads to another parking area; an equestrian trail marked with red diamonds crosses. Stay with the orange blazes of the **Florida Trail,** walking past a sign that says TRAIL. The fall colors of the floodplain forest dance off to the left. As the trail heads due east, the cedars get thicker and thicker throughout the understory of the palm hammock as the elevation drops a little, bringing dark earth underfoot and tunnels of wax myrtles heavy with berries. If you hear a distant buzz, it's likely airboat tours on the St. Johns River.

Stepping out into the sun for the first time on this hike at 1.5 miles, you see a touch of color on the sweetgum trees as you glance over and see the power lines on the right-hand side. The trail emerges along a marsh before crossing Power Line Road at another trailhead, continuing across a bridge over the canal on the south side of the road. Entering a palm hammock with ancient live oaks, where a palm arcs over the trail, you can see the floodplain of the St. Johns River crowding close off to the left. In this maze of cabbage palms, pay attention for the blazes, as the understory is very open.

At 2.3 miles, you reach the intersection of yellow, blue, and orange blazes with a sign for Tiger Branch 2.8 miles to the south. Turn left to follow the blue blazes to take a quick peek down the Swamp Spur. The trail narrows down quickly and slips between a wonderland of cypress knees in all sorts of fantastical shapes. These ancient cypresses have deeply fluted bases. Beware of the deep mud holes close to the creek near the TRAIL END sign. Retrace your steps back to the trail junction and turn left, following the orange and yellow blazes toward Tiger Creek. After crossing an old forest road, the trail climbs up and over a small berm into a palm and oak hammock, where you'll walk beneath an enormous cedar en route to the next maze of palms.

As the trail gains a little elevation, it rises into a forest of pines and oaks, where the footpath is now wonderfully carpeted with pine needles, as is every inch of the forest floor, burying the understory plants and grasses. At 3.1 miles, cross a small creek on a series of concrete steps; blue flag iris blooms here in spring. Meandering through a mature pine forest, the trail turns down a straightaway of wax myrtle and saw palmetto before entering a corridor of young cabbage palms, one of the most beautiful palm hammocks along this hike. The footpath rises out of the palm hammock and into pine/palm flatwoods before crossing a grassy forest road. At the next trail junction, 4.2 miles into your hike, the **Yellow Trail** turns north and leaves the route you're following. If you've had to wade any of the hike thus far, use this trail to cut the overall hike route to less than 8 miles. Otherwise, turn left to follow the orange blazes of the **Florida Trail** south.

The footpath emerges into open pine flatwoods with a grassy understory, perfect for deer to browse. The pines are quite old, tall and spindly. A cypress swamp parallels off to the left. The trail crosses a forest road at a double blaze, and you find a most unusual bridge made of a telephone pole with crosspieces that look like ladder rungs. Dropping down into a marshy area, the trail zigzags and enters a young forest, a restoration area. It can be difficult to follow the blazes, and impossible to find the footpath. Keep alert. By 5.5 miles you reach a sign (which points in the opposite direction) for the Tiger Branch Campsite. This is a great place to stop for lunch. Follow the blue blazes to the campsite, which has a large picnic table under the pines.

Returning to the main trail, turn left. You'll head southwest briefly before reaching the next trail junction. Here, at 6 miles, the **Florida Trail** goes west, with a small sign for JIM CREEK. To make it back to your car before dark, turn right to follow the **White Trail,**

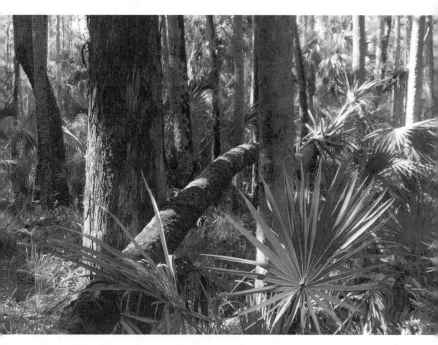

DENSE HYDRIC HAMMOCK AT TOSOHATCHEE WMA

blazed white. The trail crosses a parking area along Fish Hole Road and crosses a ditch on a bridge to enter the pine woods on the other side. As you walk along the **White Trail** through the pines, the stillness is absolute, the sense of solitude certain. This is one of the lesser-used trails in the preserve, and it shows in the lack of trail maintenance. You may frequently find yourself pushing through dense saw palmetto fronds along this section, and continually watching for the next white blaze. The trail stays atop a low berm that once served as a narrow-gauge logging railroad bed. At 6.5 miles the trail drops off the berm into a thicket of saw palmetto, skimming along the edges of wet prairies. A stand of ancient saw palmetto attempts to mimic the cabbage palms of this forest, their skinny trunks rising nearly 10 feet high. As saw palmetto grows barely an inch a year, it takes a long time for a thicket like this to form. Just beyond the thicket is a rusted piece of rail from the old railroad, and you're following its tracks once again.

As you're swimming through saw palmetto fronds, looking for the next white blaze, notice that the tall slash pines are especially old and spindly overhead, providing little shade. By 7.1 miles, you reach the intersection with the incoming **Yellow Trail,** with a sign pointing to Tiger Branch Campsite. Cross this junction and continue straight ahead. The going gets much easier. The trail passes through patches of prairie in the pine flatwoods, and it's here you'll find some of the prettiest wildflowers along the trail, including brilliant orange pine lilies in the summer months. Working its way into a denser understory, the trail continues through the pines. After crossing a bridge to a forest road, the trail leaves this road off to the left at an angle and heads down an old tramway. Lance-leaved arrowhead and other aquatic plants are briefly underfoot before the trail rises into the slightly wet flatwoods, where coreopsis puts on a show with its yellow blooms against the haze of wiregrass. Keep alert to the twists and turns of the trail through these open flatwoods. You emerge at the back side of a sign that says TRAIL at 8.4 miles. Turn right and follow the grassy strip to Power Line Road. Cross it and continue through

Parking Area 26. Immediately after crossing the tree line, the trail makes a sharp left, tacking away from where you expect to go. Tunneling deep into palm hammocks again, the trail demands that you keep watch for the next blaze in this open understory. Marsh ferns crowd close to the footpath.

By 9.5 miles, you reach the northernmost junction of trails. The **White Trail** heads left toward the main entrance of Tosohatchee WMA. The orange blazes of the **Florida Trail** come in from the north and head southeast toward where your car is parked. Turn right and head down this forest road for 0.3 mile, keeping alert for orange blazes at a FLORIDA TRAIL sign. It doesn't take long to enter the palm hammocks again, where roots and soft earth can trip up tired feet. The trail winds its way through a swampy place around the large, buttressed bases of cypress trees. A bright patch becomes obvious to the right, sun drenching the edge of the forest from the clearing along Power Line Road. It's time to watch for that blue blaze back to the parking area. Turn right and walk out to the parking area, wrapping up this all-day traverse at 11.7 miles.

Nearby Attractions

Just east of Christmas, along FL 50, A-Awesome Airboat Rides departs from the St. Johns River bridge to take you on a spin along the fringe of Tosohatchee: **airboatride.com.** En route, you'll pass Florida's largest alligator—200 feet long—and a bit of roadside whimsy that makes up the entrance to Jungle Adventures Nature Park, an alligator farm with a conservation twist: **jungleadventures.com.**

Directions

Follow FL 50 east from Orlando to Christmas. Past the post office, turn right on Taylor Creek Road. Continue 2.8 miles to the preserve entrance. Turn left. Follow Power Line Road. Drive to the parking area at the corner of Fishhole Road and Power Line Road. The trailhead parking is on the north side of Power Line Road.

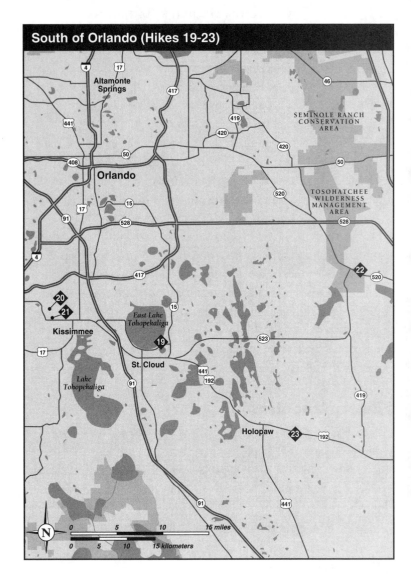

South of Orlando (Hikes 19-23)

South

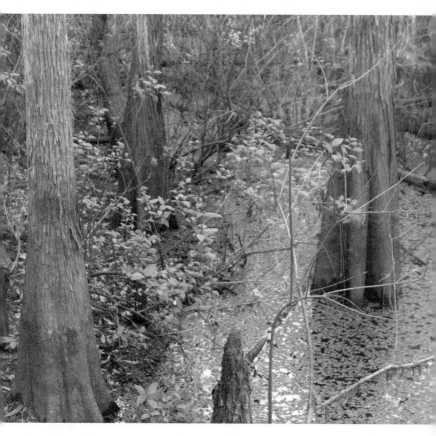

CYPRESS SWAMP

19 Lake Runnymede Conservation Area

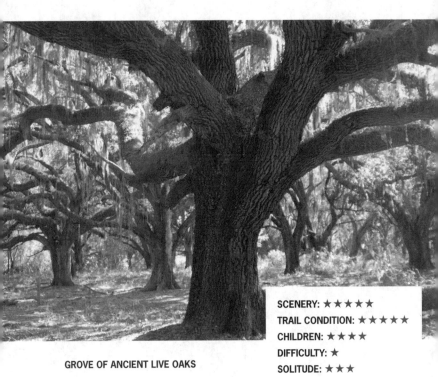

GROVE OF ANCIENT LIVE OAKS

SCENERY: ★ ★ ★ ★ ★
TRAIL CONDITION: ★ ★ ★ ★ ★
CHILDREN: ★ ★ ★ ★
DIFFICULTY: ★
SOLITUDE: ★ ★

GPS TRAILHEAD COORDINATES: N28° 35.258' W81° 09.353'

DISTANCE & CONFIGURATION: 0.9-mile double loop

HIKING TIME: 45 minutes

HIGHLIGHTS: Ancient live oaks, birding, views of East Lake Tohopekaliga

ACCESS: Free; open daily, sunrise–sunset

MAPS: USGS *St. Cloud North*

FACILITIES: Composting privy, picnic tables and grills, group campsite

WHEELCHAIR ACCESS: None

COMMENTS: No running water

CONTACTS: Osceola County Environmental Lands (407) 742-8650; **osceola.org/parks
/home.cfm**

Overview

Lake Runnymede Conservation Area is only 43 acres, but what a pre-serve! Sandwiched between the massive East Lake Tohopekaliga and the much smaller Lake Runnymede, it showcases one of the most spectacular stands of ancient live oaks in Central Florida. This short hike has a true Old South feel, with Spanish moss swaying in the breeze in thick draperies from the limbs of enormous live oaks.

Route Details

As you enter the preserve gate from the parking lot, two hiking loops start from this point, the green-blazed **Live Oak Trail** and the yellow-blazed **Lake Trail.** Turn right to take a look at the kiosk and map and to start the **Lake Trail.** Following this trail, you are beneath a dense can-opy of live oaks laden with Spanish moss. Markers guide you along the path. At the first junction, turn right. The footpath parallels Rum-mell Road, and you can see the glimmering waters of East Lake Toho-pekaliga through the residences on the other side of the road. Passing a bench, you see a cross-shaped impression of an ancient oak that was lopped off at the surface, probably after falling over. The bases of these live oaks are enormous, their age easily 500 years or more.

Passing under the arching limb of a live oak, the trail drops down past historic cattle pens (hearkening to St. Cloud's ranching heritage) and hangs a right. Snaking beneath more live oaks, the trail emerges into an open stretch of bright-white sand, a scrub between smaller oaks. Tacking to the right, turning to the left, the trail works its way into another shady stand of oaks near the road. One oak on the left is particularly massive in size, its limbs about two-thirds the breadth of the trunk itself. The trail curves out of this stand of oaks past a partially fallen one, half its trunk settled down into the sand of the scrub.

While the footpath follows the shoreline of Lake Runnymede, the water is not visible because there is too much vegetation in the way. After 0.5 mile, the trail comes up to a picnic table, with a giant

Lake Runnymede Conservation Area

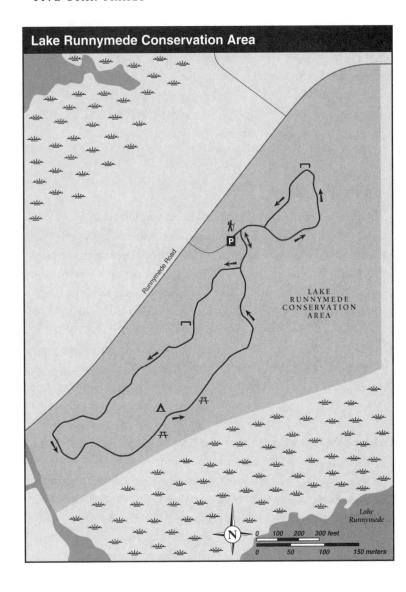

LAKE
RUNNYMEDE
CONSERVATION
AREA

Runnymede Road

Lake
Runnymede

0   100   200   300 feet

0   50   100   150 meters

N

bromeliad dangling in the branches above. The trail tacks to the right past a fire ring, a wood grill, and another picnic table, all part of the group campsite. Posts lead you through the open area. Getting out of the sun quickly, you enter another beauty spot under the oaks with more picnic tables and barbecue grills.

Songbirds, including cardinals and titmouse, flutter between the trees as you zigzag back and forth along the footpath. The trail makes a quick left through a patch of shade and ducks beneath live oaks with limbs so low they tempt tree climbers. By 0.7 mile, you return to the main entrance and its solar-powered privy. Walk past it and continue along the green-blazed **Live Oak Trail**. This heads into another portion of the live oak forest.

The loop begins quickly, with an arrow pointing to the left. The oaks are dense enough that you can't see the nearby road. They are younger than those on the other loop but still easily more than a century or two old. A tall slash pine rises to the right. You may hear the creel of a red-shouldered hawk or see its shadow as it glides overhead. Past a bench on the left, the trail curves to the right and down an elegant alley framed by the live oaks. There is a grassy prairie off to the left as you curve around to the right to finish this small loop. Turn left to exit to the parking area, completing this 0.9-mile stroll.

Nearby Attractions

Continue west along Rummell Road to Lakeshore Boulevard to access St. Cloud Lakefront Park, which features several miles of paved urban trail along the shores of East Lake Tohopekaliga, anchored by a marina, restaurant, and fishing pier.

Directions

From Florida's Turnpike, Kissimmee/St. Cloud exit, follow US 192/441 east for 4.6 miles to Orange Avenue. Turn left. Continue 1.1 miles to Rummell Road. Turn right. Lake Runnymede Conservation Area is on the right after 0.4 mile.

20 # Shingle Creek Regional Park: Historic Babb Landing

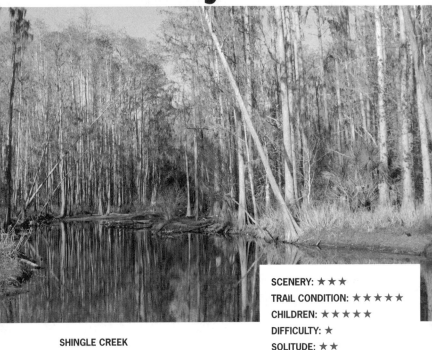

SHINGLE CREEK

SCENERY: ★ ★ ★
TRAIL CONDITION: ★ ★ ★ ★ ★
CHILDREN: ★ ★ ★ ★ ★
DIFFICULTY: ★
SOLITUDE: ★ ★

GPS TRAILHEAD COORDINATES: N28° 19.088' W81° 27.433'

DISTANCE & CONFIGURATION: 1.8-mile balloon

HIKING TIME: 1 hour

HIGHLIGHTS: Shingle Creek and historic homestead

ACCESS: Free; open daily, sunrise–sunset

MAPS: USGS *Kissimmee*

FACILITIES: Composting privy, picnic tables, playground, horseshoe pit

WHEELCHAIR ACCESS: Fully accessible

COMMENTS: Leashed pets welcome

CONTACTS: Osceola County Parks & Recreation (407) 742-7800; **osceola.org/parks
/home.cfm**

Overview

Most notable as the northernmost waterway feeding the Everglades ecosystem—via the Kissimmee River and Lake Okeechobee— Shingle Creek rises from wetlands in a part of Orlando now nearly paved over by hotels and attractions, a watershed buried by the bustle of International Drive. In pioneer times, Shingle Creek was an important link for settlers to the civilized world in Kissimmee, so numerous homesteads once edged the waterway, such as this one at Historic Babb Landing.

Route Details

Leaving the parking area by using the sidewalk, walk up past the historic homestead to the trail kiosk. As you head down the **Shingle Creek Heritage Trail,** notice its unusual, undulating but firm surface, like recycled concrete. You will see horseshoe pits off to the right, adjoining the historic structures. An inviting playground off to the left beckons youngsters to its climbing and bouncing structures and big sandbox. At the trail junction, turn right. You'll see trail markers with mileage, but they don't correspond to this route. On the right are large live oaks shading a picnic table. A line of cypresses in the distance straight ahead marks where Shingle Creek flows through the park.

At the next intersection, there is a bench and a tipped-over live oak; the orange grove is to your right and a boardwalk to the left. Turn right to follow the main trail as it parallels Shingle Creek. You pass a copse of oaks with ornamental palms growing beneath them. To the left is a broad field of dog fennel, the flat ground stretching down to the floodplain of the creek, snags providing perches for osprey and hawks to watch activity along the creek.

After 0.5 mile, there is a trail junction with a massive live oak on the left, its crown spread shading a picnic table. A broad boardwalk leads down to the banks of Shingle Creek. Slow-moving but clear, the creek threads its way between cypress-lined banks upstream to

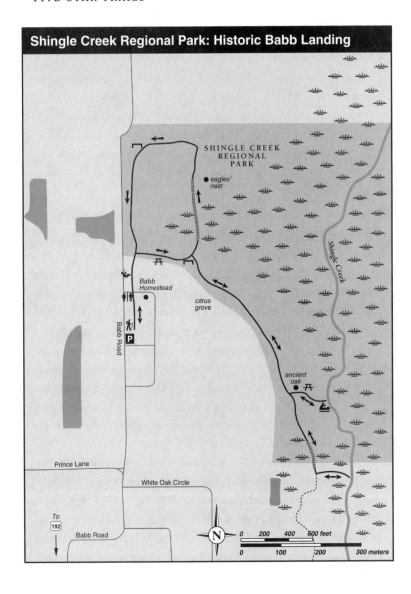

Shingle Creek Regional Park: Historic Babb Landing

flow gently between the cypresses and red maples downstream. A blue marker here indicates the start of the blue-blazed paddling trail that connects this park and the Historic Steffee Homestead (Hike 21, page 141). Fish dart through the water, and alligators may rest in the shallows. The footprints of raccoons decorate the soft muck of the creek bank. Despite the wilderness feel of the waterway, the closeness of urban life intrudes with sirens, horns, and traffic noises from nearby US 192.

Turn around and head back to the junction at the large oak tree, and turn left to continue along the trail. Cross another large, broad boardwalk over an ephemeral stream. Make a left at this next junction. A rusting barbed wire fence marks part of the old homestead between the path and the tributary. It just takes a few moments to reach Shingle Creek again, here with a different perspective. As has happened to so many Florida waterways, this portion of the creek has been turned into a canal, the sinuous nature of the swamp replaced with straight lines plowing through the landscape. A landing is on the far side of the creek.

Return to the previous trail junction, which is on the edge of a vast field of tall grass. The path straight ahead goes to another parking area, so make this your turnaround point. Turn right and continue over the ephemeral stream and back to the junction with the large oak. Bear left to follow the trail back to the junction with the fallen oak. Walk straight ahead over the boardwalk. It provides an outflow for the floodplain in times of high water. Focus your attention on the tall pines to the right as the boardwalk ends, as there is an eagles' nest. In winter and spring, both parents are present, participating in the miracle of raising a new generation. You may only see their heads bobbing up above the tall funnel of tree limbs that comprise the nest, or you might catch a glimpse of an eagle perched above, ready for the hunt.

The trail makes a sharp left turn to follow the oak-shaded property line and turns left again at a bench. This straightaway leads you right back past the playground and completes the upper loop. Continue past the historic homestead to exit, completing this 1.8-mile hike.

Nearby Attractions

Shingle Creek Regional Park is one of the closest places for an urban hike near Walt Disney World: **disneyworld.com.** Old Town, a popular shopping and entertainment complex, is along US 192 West: **myold townusa.com.** And just 1.4 miles south is another entry in this book, Shingle Creek Regional Park: Historic Steffee Homestead (Hike 21, page 141).

Directions

From I-4, Exit 68 at Downtown Disney, follow FL 535 (Vineland Road) south for 3.6 miles to US 192; turn left. Drive east on US 192 for 2.7 miles to Old Vineland Road; turn left. After 0.5 mile, turn right at the fork onto Babb Road. Follow it for 0.6 mile to where it ends at the parking area.

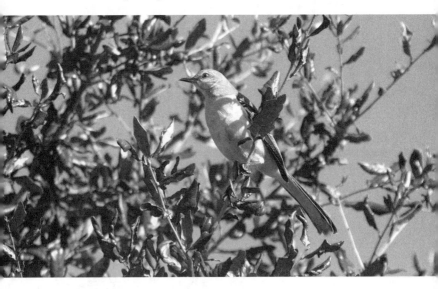

GRAY CATBIRD

Shingle Creek Regional Park: Historic Steffee Homestead

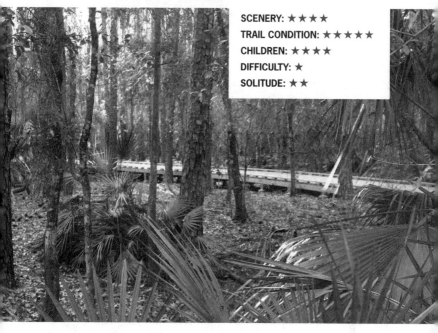

SCENERY: ★ ★ ★ ★
TRAIL CONDITION: ★ ★ ★ ★ ★
CHILDREN: ★ ★ ★ ★
DIFFICULTY: ★
SOLITUDE: ★ ★

BOARDWALK THROUGH PINE LOWLANDS

GPS TRAILHEAD COORDINATES: N28° 18.206' W81° 27.185'

DISTANCE & CONFIGURATION: 1.3-mile balloon

HIKING TIME: 1 hour

HIGHLIGHTS: Historic homestead and extensive boardwalks

ACCESS: Free; open daily, sunrise–sunset

MAPS: USGS *Kissimmee*

FACILITIES: Picnic tables and benches, composting privy, interpreted historic sites

WHEELCHAIR ACCESS: Fully accessible

COMMENTS: Leashed pets welcome

CONTACTS: Osceola County Parks & Recreation (407) 742-7800; **osceola.org/parks /home.cfm**

Shingle Creek Regional Park: Historic Steffee Homestead

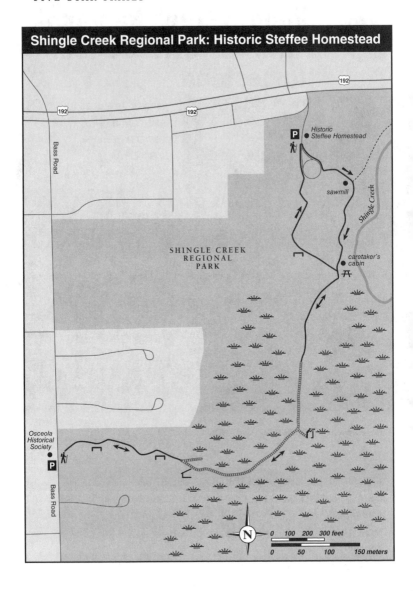

Overview

Shingle Creek is the northernmost tributary feeding Lake Okeechobee and the Everglades. On its southward flow, toward Lake Tohopekaliga, it winds through what is now some of the densest urban mass in Central Florida. Still, Shingle Creek Regional Park preserves more than 450 acres along its banks, including the Historic Steffee Homestead, a lushly forested park along US 192. With extensive boardwalks amid a cypress floodplain, it's an oasis of beauty in a busy urban corridor.

Route Details

The parking area adjoins a beautiful circa 1911 farmhouse tucked in under the canopy of old live oak trees. Trails radiate in several directions from the turnaround loop for the parking area. Head toward the picnic pavilion, where there is a restroom and a kiosk with map. From the kiosk, go straight ahead past historical farm implements and a small sawmill. Like the Historic Babb Landing site, this is another concrete trail, uneven underfoot, which winds through the forest of slash pine, oaks, and saw palmetto in the understory. As an urban park, it's busy with people walking dogs, pushing strollers, and jogging. On the left, just past the junction with an incoming trail from the right, is the caretaker's house, circa 1920. Made of cypress, it's a gorgeous piece of vernacular Florida architecture, with an open-air porch overlooking a waterway and an outdoor kitchen. Unlike the other Shingle Creek Regional Park hike (Hike 20, page 136), you never actually see the creek along this route, but you explore tributaries flowing down to the creek.

The trail continues deeper into the pine woods. Make a left at the next junction, where there is a picnic table off the trail. The concrete path grows broader to lead you through the oak and pine forest, the understory very open. Wild citrus, a legacy left from pioneer days, grows beneath a live oak's spreading crown. Passing under the large oaks, the trail continues into the floodplain and becomes a broad boardwalk. At 0.4 mile, there is a junction with a trail to the right. A platform on the left provides a place to watch for birds and look out over a sluggish cypress-lined creek that flows into Shingle Creek. Stand still and you may hear the tap-tap-tap of a downy woodpecker. From the signage, it's apparent that the boardwalk will eventually be extended farther in this direction. For now, backtrack from this observation platform and turn left to follow the boardwalk toward the Bass Road Trailhead, the back gate to this park.

As the boardwalk winds beneath the cypress trees, notice the watermarks on the tree trunks, some as high as 3 feet. Flooding can occur down Shingle Creek, as it traps an enormous amount of urban drainage. If the boardwalk is underwater, don't attempt to walk on it. Cypresses surround and shade this walk, with vast masses of marsh fern swarming around their bases. Loblolly bay, red maple, and dahoon holly lend their colorful trunks and leaves to the floodplain forest mix. Slash pines stand in tall columns against the blue sky.

After 0.5 mile, you reach a T-intersection with a boardwalk that was once part of an old nature trail. Turn right and take a peek at the detailed interpretive information down this dead-end spur before heading in the opposite direction. Passing a rain shelter, the board-walk soon ends and becomes a concrete path through the woods again, slipping between the tall pines and clumps of saw palmetto. The Bass Road Trailhead is at 0.7 mile. It is only open Thursday–Sunday, the same days that the adjacent Osceola County Histori-cal Society Pioneer Village & Museum is open, and provides a place to park. Before Shingle Creek Regional Park existed, this was the entrance to Steffee Preserve; you can see faint traces of the old nature trail through the woods. If the gate is open, consider wander-ing across the street to enjoy living history at the Pioneer Village. This is your turnaround point.

Follow the boardwalk back through the cypress floodplain. At the intersection with the observation platform boardwalk, turn left to meander along the broad boardwalk under the pines. After the boardwalk ends, you return to the spot with the creekside picnic table and caretaker's home. Turn left on this trail to walk among the saw palmetto and slash pines; a smattering of wiregrass grows beneath them. Passing a bench, you can see the park boundary fence on the left and tall saw palmetto on the right. The trail emerges at the turn-around for the parking area within sight of the Steffee Homestead farmhouse, returning you to your car at 1.3 miles.

Nearby Attractions

Shingle Creek Regional Park is one of the closest places for an urban hike near Walt Disney World: **disneyworld.com.** Outside the back gate of this park, the Osceola County Historical Society Pioneer Village & Museum provides a glimpse into the region's pioneer past, with bluegrass jams on Sundays: **osceolahistory.com.** Another entry in this book, Shingle Creek Regional Park: Historic Babb Landing (Hike 20, page 136), is 1.4 miles north.

Directions

From I-4, Exit 68 at Downtown Disney, follow FL 535 (Vineland Road) south for 3.6 miles to US 192; turn left. Drive east on US 192 for 3 miles to the entrance on the right, just past Old Vineland Road.

Taylor Creek Loop

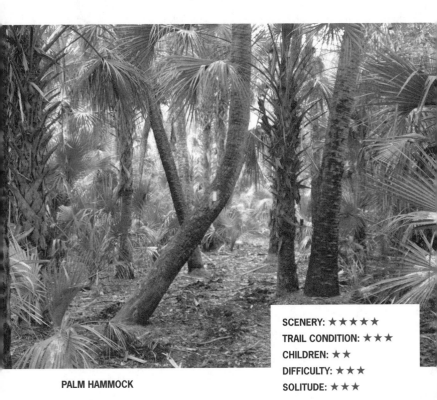

PALM HAMMOCK

SCENERY: ★ ★ ★ ★ ★
TRAIL CONDITION: ★ ★ ★
CHILDREN: ★ ★
DIFFICULTY: ★ ★ ★
SOLITUDE: ★ ★ ★

GPS TRAILHEAD COORDINATES: N28° 22.434' W80° 54.259'

DISTANCE & CONFIGURATION: 4.7-mile loop

HIKING TIME: 3 hours

HIGHLIGHTS: Palm hammocks, cypress swamp, wildflowers

ACCESS: Free; open daily, sunrise–sunset

MAPS: USGS *Lake Poinsett SW*

FACILITIES: Picnic tables

WHEELCHAIR ACCESS: None

COMMENTS: The trail floods when the St. Johns River is high. Use mosquito repellent.

CONTACTS: Florida Fish and Wildlife Conservation Commission Regional Office (352) 732-1225; **myfwc.com/viewing/recreation/wmas/lead/Tosohatchee**

Overview

An exploration into the wilderness fringe along the St. Johns River west of Cocoa, the Taylor Creek Loop immerses you in the shade of ancient palm trees in the river floodplain. Built by the Indian River chapter of the Florida Trail Association, this well-established trail remains high and dry as long as the river is within its banks. Expect a wonderland of botanical beauty along this 4.7-mile loop, truly one of Florida's best hikes to enjoy the splendor of palm hammocks.

Route Details

Starting from the east side of the parking area, the white blazes guide you right into the first palm hammock, a nice junglelike corridor with palm fronds slapping you in the face as you head downhill. Since the footpath is not well worn, be sure to keep looking for the next white blaze, or you might find yourself down a deer trail. Leaving the corridor of palms, the trail continues into wet pine flatwoods of loblolly and slash pine. Cars zoom past nearby as the trail parallels FL 520 for a short stretch, but at least you get this noisy part of the hike out of the way first. Watch for a double blaze past a couple of wetland areas where blue flag iris blooms in the spring. The trail makes a sharp right back into a palm hammock. Wild hogs have made deep burrows in the footpath, making the going tricky due to uneven terrain underfoot. Some of the cabbage palms actually look furry from a distance, thanks to the pine needles stuck in their bootjacks.

Turning away from the highway, the trail makes a soft right to head toward a hammock of very large live oaks. Draped in Spanish moss, covered in ferns and red blanket lichen, and dripping with bromeliads, these oaks are truly picturesque. However, if you spend too much time looking up, you will fall down because of the rough tread underfoot. Masses of mushy sphagnum moss appear along the trail, indicating that this area does flood at times. After 0.5 mile, the hammock becomes more majestic, with larger live oaks festooned with resurrection fern. Large goldfoot ferns drape out of the cabbage

Taylor Creek Loop

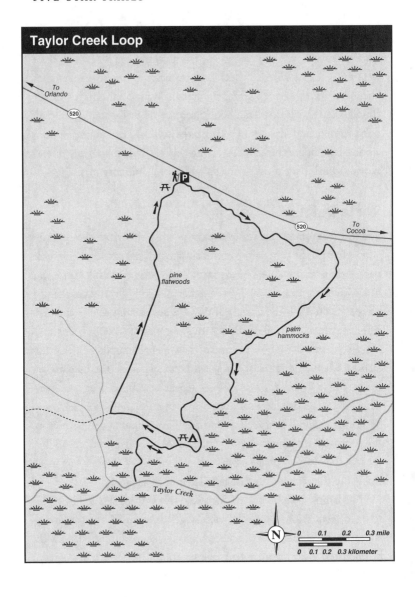

palms, and colorful American beautyberry shrubs show off their shiny purple berries throughout the understory. Entering a virtual maze of cabbage palm trunks, the deeper you get into the hammocks, the smaller you feel. The trail runs along the edge of a large marsh, hidden by a dense fringe of wax myrtle, with deer tracks impressed into the rich, black earth underfoot. At a large spreading live oak, thick grapevines dangle down, a few forming an odd shape like a suspended bed frame.

Walk softly as you approach a broad, duckweed-covered canal, and you may see alligators. The trail turns right, heading south. You pass a cabbage palm with a 90° bend in its trunk, leaving the highway and the canal behind to burrow deeper into the palm hammocks. The trail circles a marsh with duck potato in bloom. A little more sun filters into the canopy as you reach 1 mile. The trail continues to twist through more palm hammocks, reaching a wonderful montage of oaks, resurrection ferns, and cabbage palms with trunks crispy and singed by wildfire. Farther along, a star-shaped sphagnum moss covers the trunks of the tall palms. It feels like a carpet if you run your hand along it. The trail continues to zigzag through mazes of palm trunks. By 1.9 miles, you glimpse a little horizon through the trees, the distant river floodplain, which the trail turns away from. Deep in the palm hammocks, there is dense shade, allowing colorful fungi and lichens to thrive. You reach a quiet place, with only the rustle of the cabbage palm fronds in the breeze. Clouds drift across patches of blue sky between the palms.

Cypress knees appear off to the left at 2.5 miles, signaling you're drawing near to Taylor Creek. The trail reaches a picnic table at the primitive campsite. This is also a trail junction with a spur trail down to the creek. As you walk atop the soft pine needles, the trail narrows and narrows; mosquitoes become more intense. Floodplain trees intrude into the pine forest. Turn left at the T and continue along the white blazes beneath the ancient cypresses. The closer you get to the creek, the rougher and muckier the terrain becomes, with cypress knees jutting out of the footpath. Blazes lead you right down into the cypress swamp to the TAYLOR CREEK TRAIL END sign, which might be underwater when you reach it, at 2.9 miles. Return back along the spur trail to the trail junction. Turn left.

White blazes now guide you down a forest road, a broad walkway through the pine flatwoods. A stand of silver-tinged saw palmetto sits to the side as you approach a sign at 3.6 miles, marking where the trail turns to the right. Notice the gentle elevation gain and colorful wildflowers, such as bachelor's button. Songbirds trill from the pines. Passing several ephemeral wetlands, the road curves through the forest, gently guiding you back to a cable gate and picnic table at the trailhead after 4.7 miles.

Nearby Attractions

A longtime landmark along the St. Johns River, Lone Cabbage Fish Camp shouldn't be missed. Enjoy funky waterfront dining, live music, and airboat rides into the expansive marshes of the river: **twisterair boatrides.com/cabbage.htm.**

Directions

Taylor Creek Loop is located along FL 520 between FL 528 and FL 524, 2 miles west of the St. Johns River on the south side of the highway. Since this stretch of highway has a high fence, be alert for a gate with an "FT" symbol on it. If you're approaching from I-95 in Cocoa, it's easy to find since there is a turnout, the first you'll find after crossing the St. Johns River. Open the unlocked gate to enter the trailhead, which has ample parking and picnic tables. Be sure to close the gate to protect wildlife from high-speed traffic.

23

Triple N Ranch Wildlife Management Area

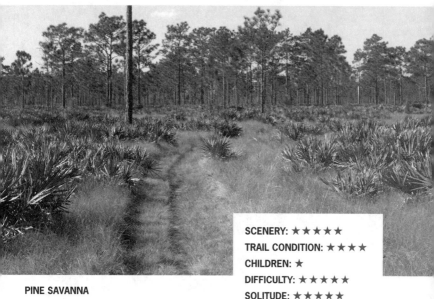

SCENERY: ★ ★ ★ ★ ★
TRAIL CONDITION: ★ ★ ★ ★
CHILDREN: ★
DIFFICULTY: ★ ★ ★ ★ ★
SOLITUDE: ★ ★ ★ ★ ★

PINE SAVANNA

GPS TRAILHEAD COORDINATES: N28° 07.827' W81° 01.227'

DISTANCE & CONFIGURATION: 7.5-mile loop

HIKING TIME: 5½–8 hours, depending on water levels

HIGHLIGHTS: Vast pine savannas, pitcher plant bogs, cypress floodplain swamp

ACCESS: Free; open daily, sunrise–sunset

MAPS: USGS *Holopaw, Holopaw SE,* and *Deer Park*

FACILITIES: Composting privy at trailhead and a picnic table

WHEELCHAIR ACCESS: None

COMMENTS: This is one of Florida's most physically demanding hikes, especially if there is water in the floodplain. Allow plenty of daylight to complete the loop. As this is a hunting preserve, check hunt dates before setting out: **myfwc.com.** There is also open range here, so be alert for cattle.

CONTACTS: Florida Fish and Wildlife Conservation Commission Regional Office (352) 732-1225; **myfwc.com/viewing/recreation/wmas/lead/triple-n-ranch**

Triple N Ranch Wildlife Management Area

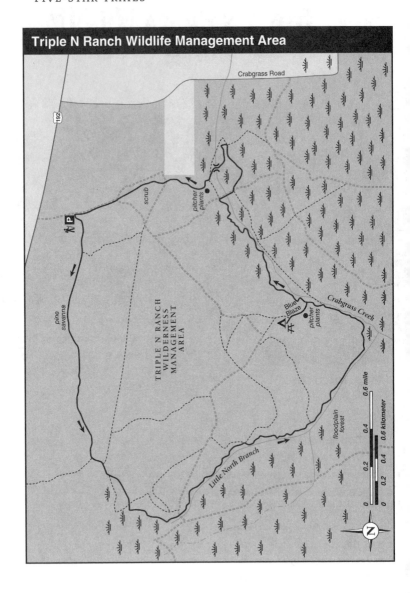

Overview

With a rugged but well-marked loop trail traversing landscapes both panoramic and intimate, Triple N Ranch Wildlife Management Area (WMA) protects more than 16,000 acres of wide-open pine savanna, grassy prairies, cypress domes, and the cypress-lined floodplain of Crabgrass Creek. Surrounded by some of Florida's largest cattle ranches, it is a haven for both wildlife and botanical beauty, with extensive pitcher plant bogs, ancient oaks and cypresses, and colorful pine flatwoods wildflowers. With the 7.3-mile loop trail clambering in and out of the creek floodplain for more than half the route, this is a very strenuous backcountry adventure.

Route Details

The trail starts just beyond the hunt camp campground at a kiosk. Sign in before you head out into the backcountry of this preserve. As you follow the trail west, look down at your feet. You'll see yellow-eyed grass, sundews, and wild bachelor's button—a few of the many wildflowers you'll find along this hike. The hike begins amid the vastness of the Great Osceola Pine Savanna, an immense landscape of prairie grasses dotted with longleaf pine. Straight ahead, it's broken up by a handful of cypress domes. By 0.4 mile, you're immersed in the open pine savanna, a habitat that William Bartram once described as covering much of the uplands of Florida.

A thicket of saw palmetto grows waist- to shoulder-high, and the trail weaves through it beneath the tall, scattered long-leaf pines. Listen for the sounds of red-cockaded woodpeckers, an endangered species that thrives around these ancient pines, which the birds use for nesting. Deer trails crisscross open patches of prairie grasses. The bright line of a cypress strand is evident on the right, beyond the pines. As you draw close to another cypress dome at 1.5 miles, the trail reaches a T-intersection with a forest road. Turn left. At the next set of double blazes at the fork, keep right. Crossing another forest road at 1.6 miles, you see beehives off to the right. The trail narrows to head toward the outline of a creek defined by cabbage palms and cypresses. The shallow waterway may be dry as you step across its small impression in the landscape and climb out of the creek basin into a grassy prairie with flat-topped goldenrod. Crossing an old forest road at 1.9 miles, follow the quartet of blazes as they curve the trail left into a hardwood hammock past a gathering of bladderworts. This is the first serious patch of shade along the trail, which explains the number of cow patties beneath the trees.

Popping out into the sun along the line of trees, the trail passes painted-out blazes that lead into the pine flatwoods. At 2.2 miles, the trail dives into a dense thicket of saw palmetto to enter the floodplain of Little Crabgrass Creek. Wild coffee grows throughout the understory, and shoelace fern dangles from mossy cabbage palm trunks. The corridor is not broad; you can see pine savanna in the distance in both directions. It is deeply shaded here; anything not covered by water is covered by moss. This wild, wet place is only the start of several hours of hiking in this rugged habitat. When water flows through the channel, it does so with some speed. The trail climbs out of the floodplain basin and onto the edge of the pine savanna. You reach a T junction with a former incoming trail, the blazes marked out to the left. Turn right and you soon find the sign for **Cathi's Trail,** dedicated to Cathi Riley, a longtime Florida Trail Association member who inspired this tough hike.

The trail climbs back out of the basin to the edge of the pine savanna, but only for a moment before it heads back into the shade of the floodplain of Little Crabgrass Creek. It's not easy going, between the roots and rough terrain underfoot and the spiderwebs overhead. There are pits of water off to the right before the trail makes a left turn into a drainage area. Mounds of ferns surround the footpath, and you encounter some thick mud at a creek crossing with flowing water. You emerge on the edge of the savanna and reach a T-intersection with a forest road at 3.4 miles. Turn right and follow the sandy road into the hammock. Be cautious at the next intersection, where the trail doubles back on itself around a horse-shoe in the creek; there are gaping, ankle-snatching holes along the bluff. The floodplain basin broadens where the waters of Little Crabgrass Creek and Crabgrass Creek merge. Just the slightest bit of water in this part of the floodplain results in boot-sucking mud, making for slow going.

By 4 miles, the trail climbs out of the wet zone again and is firmly in a deeply shaded palm hammock before dropping down to the floodplain again, this time beneath trees of enormous stature and a smattering of wild grapefruit. At 4.5 miles, a sign and blue blaze guide you to high ground for a break at a picnic table. As it climbs out of the floodplain, the trail is surrounded by clumps of pitcher plants on both sides of the trail. Relax at the old picnic table under the oaks before returning to the loop. Continuing counterclockwise along the loop, the trail makes another sharp horseshoe turn facing

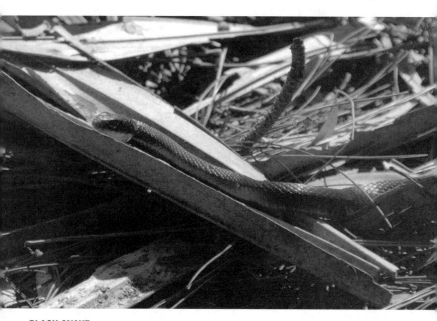

BLACK SNAKE

a forest of cypress knees and stumps along an arm of the creek. Keep watching for the next blaze as you pass under a massive red maple. Young southern magnolia and tall hickory grow along the slopes of the creek. Hopping across a small tributary, the trail winds deeper into the forest; the palm-lined creek becomes much wider as you enter a maze of cypress knees at 5.6 miles. Crossing another squishy cypress-lined corridor, the trail reaches the corner of a barbed wire fence before rising up into the pine savanna, reaching the other end of **Cathi's Trail**, marked with a sign at 5.9 miles.

Reaching an intersection with the yellow-blazed trail at a forest road, turn right. Orange and yellow blazes lead you across Crabgrass Creek over a culvert to emerge in pine uplands. Turn left. The trail meanders down a forest road through the longleaf pine forest, your first dry habitat in a while. At a T-intersection with a post wrapped in barbed wire, turn left to drop back down into the floodplain. It's tricky here as the trail heads out into the swamp. Pick the best path between the blazes. It's a relief to see a bridge to cross back over Crabgrass Creek at 6.6 miles.

Passing eight blazes (four orange, four yellow) on a single cabbage palm trunk, the trail makes a sharp left to rise out of the floodplain forest for the last time. A bonanza of pitcher plants lines the trail as you climb up into scrubby flatwoods and open scrub with bright-white sand underfoot. Turn left at the forest road. The trail makes a sharp right almost immediately as it meets the white- and yellow-blazed trails, following a line of blaze posts to higher ground. By 7 miles, you can see a collection of buildings in the distance to the right and flashes of traffic straight ahead along US 192. The trail reaches a T-intersection and turns left. Emerging at the main road through the preserve by 7.3 miles, turn right. Follow it back to the trailhead, completing this satisfying but strenuous 7.5-mile loop. Don't forget to sign out before you leave.

Nearby Attractions

Forever Florida, an ecodestination south along US 441 at Holopaw, offers guided ecosafaris, trail rides, zip lines, and canopy walks through wilderness similar to what's seen on this hike: **foreverflorida.com.**

Directions

From Kissimmee/St. Cloud, follow US 192 east toward Melbourne. Continue 3.6 miles past the turnoff for US 441 south at Holopaw to the preserve entrance on the right.

West of Orlando (Hikes 24-27)

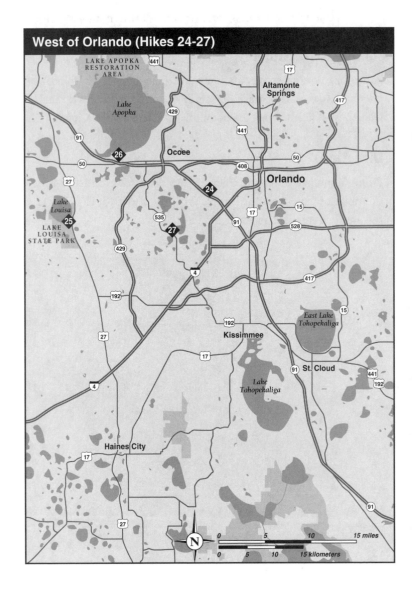

LAKE APOPKA RESTORATION AREA

Lake Apopka

Altamonte Springs

441

17

417

429

441

91

50

Ocoee

50

408

Orlando

27

535

17

15

Lake Louisa

LAKE LOUISA STATE PARK

429

91

528

24

25

26

27

4

417

192

27

East Lake Tohopekaliga

15

192

Kissimmee

17

St. Cloud

91

441

192

Lake Tohopekaliga

4

Haines City

17

91

27

0   5   10   15 miles

N

0   5   10   15 kilometers

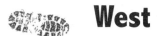

West

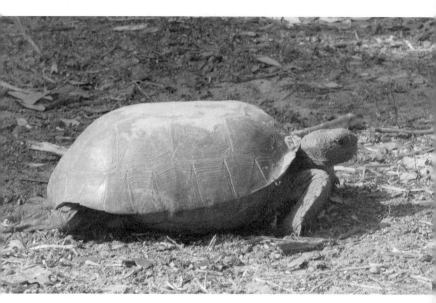

GOPHER TORTOISE

Bill Frederick Park at Turkey Lake

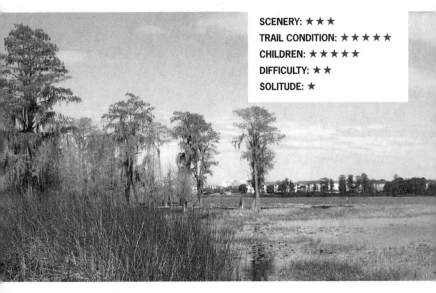

SCENERY: ★ ★ ★
TRAIL CONDITION: ★ ★ ★ ★ ★
CHILDREN: ★ ★ ★ ★ ★
DIFFICULTY: ★ ★
SOLITUDE: ★

TURKEY LAKE

GPS TRAILHEAD COORDINATES: N28° 30.021' W81° 28.503'

DISTANCE & CONFIGURATION: 2.4-mile loop

HIKING TIME: 1.5 hours

HIGHLIGHTS: Wildlife sightings, views of Turkey Lake

ACCESS: $2 per individual or $4 for vehicles with multiple passengers; November–March: daily, 8 a.m.–5 p.m.; April–October: daily, 8 a.m.–7 p.m.

MAPS: USGS *Orlando West;* cityoforlando.net/fpr/Html/PDFs/BFP_Map.pdf

FACILITIES: Extensive, including restrooms, picnic tables with grills, campground, and cabins

WHEELCHAIR ACCESS: Partial

COMMENTS: Busy on weekends. Leashed dogs are welcome but must be registered at the gate on their first visit.

CONTACTS: Bill Frederick Park at Turkey Lake (407) 246-4486; cityoforlando.net/fpr/Html/Parks/BillFrederick.htm

Overview

Long known as Turkey Lake Park, the City of Orlando's largest park covers 178 acres of rolling hills on the western shore of the lake. It's an urban complex for outdoor recreation of all sorts. Visitors come for boating on the lake and swimming in the pool. They come to picnic, to fish from the piers, to play 18-hole golf or disc golf. They come to explore the farm and observe the farm animals. They come for cabin-, tent-, and RV camping. And they come for hiking! A natural-surface nature trail runs the length of the park on its western edge. Combined with the paved bicycle path that loops the park, you can explore the entire park on this 2.4-mile walk.

Route Details

Leaving the parking area adjoining the cabins, walk toward the cabins and keep to their left, heading uphill on the grassy slope into the slash pines. A **Nature Trail** sign guides you forward toward the tree line at the top of the hill. You hear the constant hum of Florida's Turnpike, which defines the western edge of the park. Look for a small opening between the trees and a sign where the footpath begins, tunneling into sand pine scrub on this high, dry ridge above the lake. Green strands of smilax, also known as catbrier, dangle across the stunted oaks and silk bay. This trail, although close to traffic noise, has some rugged elevation gains and drops, enough to make the walk a lot of fun.

The white sand curves down into a bowl of saw palmetto before heading down a straightaway through the scrub. Passing a large pavilion above a tee for the disc golf, the trail reaches its first interpretive markers about the plants around you, such as sand pine and dahoon holly. Sand live oaks form archways over the trail. You see a disc golf hole off to the right before the trail emerges behind the Children's Farm. The trail drops down sharply before it starts to follow the fence around the big red barn. This is not a petting farm but a working farm, a great place for urban residents to bring their kids to learn

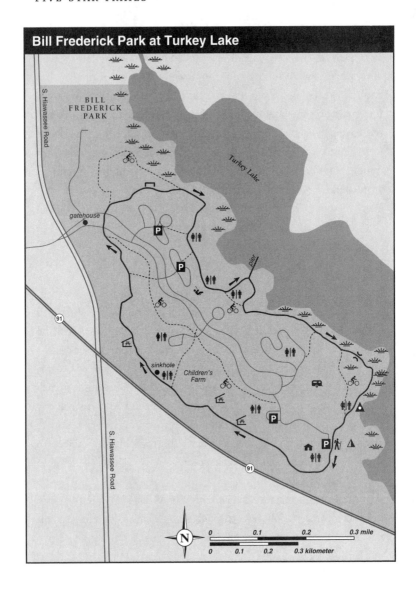

Bill Frederick Park at Turkey Lake

BILL
FREDERICK
PARK

Turkey Lake

gatehouse

pier

sinkhole

*Children's
Farm*

S. Hiawassee Road

S. Hiawassee Road

91

91

N

0   0.1   0.2   0.3 mile

0   0.1   0.2   0.3 kilometer

about farm animals. A restroom sits at the top of the hill, and there is a water fountain and bench down on the farm.

Past the farm, the trail curves around a sinkhole and a tall sand pine with an unusual split trunk. The footpath undulates up and down these ancient sand dunes, with uphill climbs. Beyond an old pavilion, the trail leaves the scrub to enter the more developed portion of the park. Watch for arrows to keep you on the trail. When you come to a junction with a bark-chip path amid the grasses, follow it to the left. It skirts between cabbage palms and oaks, passing gopher tortoise burrows. Keep left at the junction of bark-chip paths. Citrus trees, primarily kumquats, surround the trail, dripping with fruits during the winter months. Passing the **Nature Trail** sign on the left, the trail emerges at a pavilion within sight of the front gate, where there is a water fountain and benches. You've walked 1 mile.

To continue the loop, turn left on the paved bike path and cross the park road. Be alert to bicycle riders zipping past as the trail drops down a hillside of pines and oaks. Descending to Turkey Lake through the woods, you get the first glimpse of the wall-to-wall development on the far shore. Despite the crowding of civilization, the shoreline of the lake is marshy, attracting flotillas of coots drifting across the waters. The trail curves around a picnic area with covered pavilions and grills and toward a boat launch before climbing uphill past the swimming and volleyball complex. Turn left at the T-intersection.

By 1.5 miles you reach the playgrounds. Walk downhill to the pier, passing the restrooms. The pier provides a nice perspective on the near shoreline. As you leave the pier, follow the paved path up and around to the T-intersection, and make a left. Thick with cattails and pickerelweed, the next little cove is always busy with bird life. The trail continues past it, behind the campground. Turn off the paved path at pole 6 of the disc golf course to follow the lay of the land as it slopes down to a bridge. Keep alert for golfers, alligators, and ant beds as you traverse this section, passing an ancient cypress stump, and walk along the extremely marshy shoreline for a short stretch. There are benches here for wildlife-watching.

As you approach the dock, climb uphill to the bike path. You can see and hear the busy turnpike in the distance. Atop the hill, Southlake Overlook provides one more sweeping view of Turkey Lake. Returning to the bike path, walk past the ball field to return to the parking area, completing the 2.4-mile loop.

Nearby Attractions

Bill Frederick Park at Turkey Lake is less than 4 miles north of Universal Orlando (**universalorlando.com**) and 8.8 miles north of SeaWorld Orlando (**seaworldparks.com**).

Directions

From the junction of I-4 and Florida's Turnpike, drive west on I-4 to Exit 75B and follow Kirkman Road (FL 435) north for 1.6 miles. Turn left onto Conroy Road and continue 1.5 miles. Turn right on Hiawassee Road and drive 0.9 mile to the park entrance on the right. After checking in through the front gate and paying the entrance fee, follow the park road all the way back to the Carter Center, where you'll find the turnoff to the cabins. Follow this narrow road down the hill and park in this lot. Alternatively, you can park in the Carter Center lot and walk down.

Lake Louisa State Park

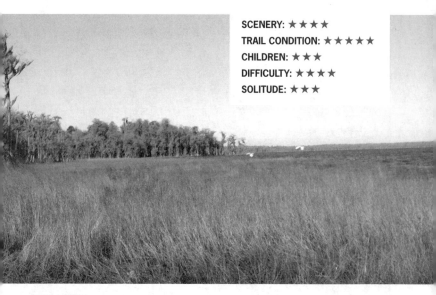

SCENERY: ★ ★ ★ ★
TRAIL CONDITION: ★ ★ ★ ★ ★
CHILDREN: ★ ★ ★
DIFFICULTY: ★ ★ ★ ★
SOLITUDE: ★ ★ ★

LAKE LOUISA

GPS TRAILHEAD COORDINATES:

Ranger Station Trailhead: N28° 27.351' W81° 43.422'

Lake Louisa Trailhead: N28° 27.630' W81° 44.856'

DISTANCE & CONFIGURATION: 4.1-mile one-way or 8.2-mile out-and-back

HIKING TIME: 3–5 hours

HIGHLIGHTS: Expansive views, shoreline of Lake Louisa

ACCESS: State park entrance fee of $2 per pedestrian or bicyclist, $4 per individual driver, $6 for 2–8 people in a vehicle; open daily, 8 a.m.–sunset

MAPS: USGS *Lake Louisa*; trail map at ranger station

FACILITIES: Restrooms at Lake Louisa Trailhead

WHEELCHAIR ACCESS: None

COMMENTS: Leashed pets welcome. Hike can be done as an out-and-back from either trailhead, doubling your mileage and time.

CONTACTS: Lake Louisa State Park (352) 394-3969; **floridastateparks.org/lakelouisa**

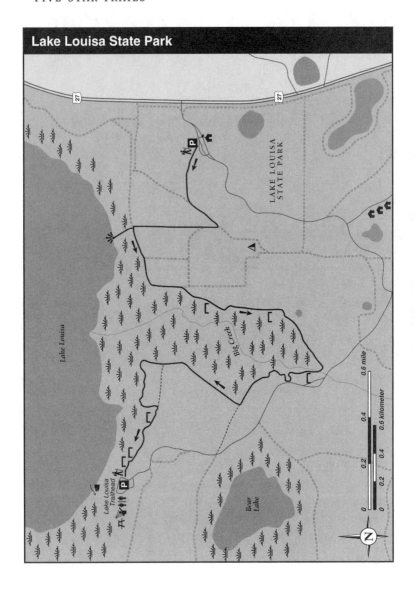

Lake Louisa State Park

Overview

In the rolling hills of the Lake Wales Ridge south of Clermont, Lake Louisa is the southernmost lake in the Palatlakaha River chain of lakes, its waters flowing northward to feed Lake Susan, Lake Minnehaha, and Lake Minneola. Formerly ranchland and orange groves atop the northernmost tip of the Lake Wales Ridge, Lake Louisa State Park is a study in restoration, as longleaf pines and wiregrass again top the high hills, and the lowlands remain thickets of hardwood forest and cypress swamps. Extending across this vertical landscape from the highest point to the lowest, the trail system immerses you in this spectrum of habitats.

Route Details

With two cars allowing you to shuttle, or a ride back from a friendly fellow camper, this hike through Lake Louisa State Park can be enjoyed as a one-way, 4.1-mile "downhill all the way" experience if you start at the parking area adjacent to the ranger station. (From there you will have a sweeping view of the lake.) There are six lakes altogether among the 4,400 acres of this park, although Louisa is the namesake and certainly the largest. When these hills were homesteaded by the Hammond family in 1910, steamboats still ran across the lake.

Turn left at the first T-intersection, your first decision point along the trail system, at 0.25 mile. The trail offers expansive views across the hillside, on which longleaf pines have a good foothold at restoring sandhill habitat. At the next T-intersection, turn right to head downhill, rounding a large marshland hidden behind a screen of vegetation on your left. Stay to the left at the next fork as the trail summits a hill and heads down the other side into the first burst of shade along the walk, a small hammock of live oak and laurel oak, as the land levels out and you reach a trail intersection.

Take a few minutes to walk straight ahead on a short spur trail that leads out to Lake Louisa. Passing through the floodplain forest that rings the lake, it scrambles over an embankment beneath a moss-draped live oak and eases down to the sandy shore. Yes, you can see houses on the far shore, but turn left and look to the cypress-lined near shore, busy with bird life. This is the only spot along the trail system where you can drink in the panorama of the natural shoreline of Lake Louisa.

Returning to the main trail, you've walked a mile so far. Turn right. The trail continues through open former pasture with a smattering of trees but no direct shade. A line of cypress is ahead in the distance. At the next trail junction, turn left as you start heading uphill, and keep right at the next fork. Passing a marsh on the left, you encounter a bench soon after as the trail works its way into some shade. Emerging back into the sun, you pass between patches of bright-white sand, which was the original scrub of the ancient Lake Wales Ridge. The trail follows a causeway through a stand of pines, before you once again come out into the sun through another open meadow that is attempting to return to scrub.

You are almost misguided into a floodplain (which isn't a problem if the creek is low) at 2.4 miles, where the trail makes its way out to the park road to enable you to cross a creek on the highway bridge. Watch for the blazes to immediately lead you back into the woods along this deeply forested waterway. This is another of the beauty spots on the trail, where the footpath guides you beneath a dense canopy of oaks as it winds along the creek before it emerges into the pine flatwoods.

Passing a junction with the fitness trail, the trail continues along the edge of a pretty little stretch of scrub up to the next trail junction at 2.7 miles. Continue straight ahead. Following a forest road that divides the former pasture/recovering scrub from the hardwoods and floodplain forest of the creek drainage, you come to a trail junction after walking across a well-used wildlife path. Turn right. Passing a bench, watch for a side trail on the right. It's a spur trail leading uphill with a bench overlooking the cypress floodplain and a small pond, another small beauty spot.

Returning to the main trail, you soon reach the eastern end of the nature trail loop. Turn right to follow this interpretive trail along the edge of the floodplain forest. It reaches a boardwalk with several benches and information about the Green Swamp watershed, of which Lake Louisa is an important part. Trails merge as you approach the trailhead kiosk at the Lake Louisa parking area at 4.1 miles. If you have arranged for a shuttle car, you've reached the end of the hike. Otherwise, return the way you came, back to the Ranger Station Trailhead, for an 8.2-mile out-and-back hike.

Nearby Attractions

Lake Louisa State Park is just 14 miles northwest of Walt Disney World: **disneyworld.com.** Head north into Clermont on US 27 to discover two Old Florida tourist attractions: the 22-story Citrus Tower (**citrustower.com**) and the adjacent Presidents Hall of Fame, a museum of Americana (**lakecountyfl.gov/hometown_highlights /presidents_hall_of_fame.aspx**).

Directions

Follow US 27 south 6.6 miles from FL 50 in Clermont to the park entrance on the right. Coming from the south, the park entrance is 8.2 miles north of US 192 along FL 27.

26

Oakland Nature Preserve

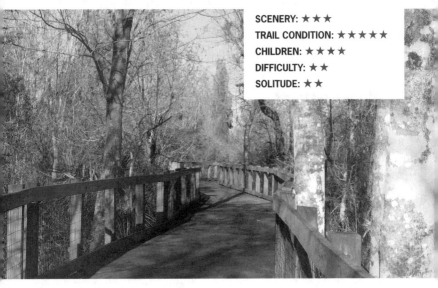

SCENERY: ★ ★ ★
TRAIL CONDITION: ★ ★ ★ ★ ★
CHILDREN: ★ ★ ★ ★
DIFFICULTY: ★ ★
SOLITUDE: ★ ★

BOARDWALK TO LAKE APOPKA

GPS TRAILHEAD COORDINATES: N28° 33.300' W81° 38.390'

DISTANCE & CONFIGURATION: 2.1-mile loop and out-and-back

HIKING TIME: 1.5 hours at a relaxed pace

HIGHLIGHTS: Sweeping view of Lake Apopka from an uncluttered shore

ACCESS: Free, but donations appreciated; open daily, 8 a.m.–sunset

MAPS: USGS *Clermont East*

FACILITIES: Nature center with restrooms and a porch with rocking chairs, access to West Orange Trail bike path

WHEELCHAIR ACCESS: The boardwalk trail is wheelchair-accessible, as is the nature center

COMMENTS: Dogs are not permitted.

CONTACTS: Oakland Nature Preserve (407) 905-0054; **oaklandnaturepreserve.org**

Overview

The trail system at Oakland Nature Preserve includes three segments you can take alone or as one hike. The boardwalk to Lake Apopka is the showcase of the preserve, offering immersion in the floodplain forest and dramatic views along the lakeshore. The Green Trail is a loop off the boardwalk through a shady oak hammock where you may see antelope or emus in the wildlife preserve next door. The Uplands Trail is a mazy network of short, hilly trails with a connection to the West Orange Trail, a major bicycle corridor.

Route Details

Along the south shore of Lake Apopka, Florida's third-largest lake, Oakland Nature Preserve protects 128 acres of natural lakefront. Part of the purpose of this preserve is to educate visitors about environmental damage done to Lake Apopka over the past century and how it is now slowly being corrected.

Start your hike by leaving the parking area to walk down to the first segment of boardwalk. Stop and sign in at the shelter. The boardwalk leads into the floodplain forest along Lake Apopka, a swamp forest dense with red maples and sweetgum trees. The boardwalk ends abruptly. The **Green Trail** goes off to the right. Keep left and follow the concrete path, which leads to the main boardwalk.

Along the broad boardwalk, the views vary according to the time of year. Floodplain forest trees showcase Florida's autumn colors, typically by December, and drop their leaves into the water, opening up broad vistas. When the trees are resplendent in greenery, the walk feels more intimate. The boardwalk makes a strong jog to the right and heads down a straightaway past tangerine trees. The uplands around Lake Apopka were once covered with citrus groves and are now crowded with subdivisions. Water sluices by quickly beneath the boardwalk in a deep cut. You reach a rain shelter after 0.25 mile.

The trail makes a curve beneath a large and colorful loblolly bay tree and passes a large dahoon holly on a small island before passing

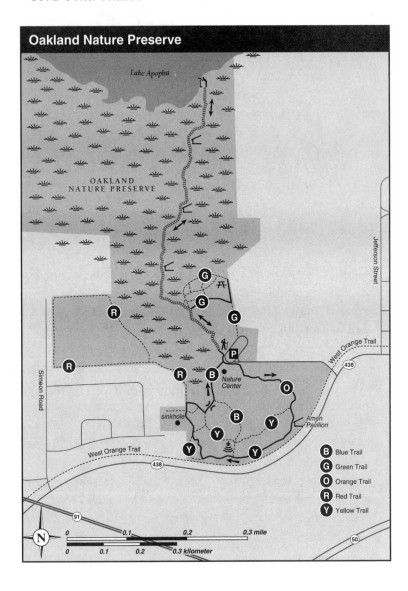

Oakland Nature Preserve

Lake Apopka

OAKLAND
NATURE PRESERVE

Jefferson Street

West Orange Trail

438

Simeon Road

Nature Center

sinkhole

Amon Pavilion

West Orange Trail

438

B Blue Trail
G Green Trail
O Orange Trail
R Red Trail
Y Yellow Trail

N

| 0 | 0.1 | 0.2 | 0.3 mile |

| 0 | 0.1 | 0.2 | 0.3 kilometer |

91

50

through another rain shelter. The swamp vegetation looks pressed down, perhaps from an alligator. The horizon line of Lake Apopka is not far off. The trail turns again, with sweeping views to the left. In the distance, a row of cabbage palms defines the far shore. The boardwalk ends at a large covered pavilion along the open water of Lake Apopka at 0.6 mile. Boaters are welcome to tie up and explore the preserve. A timeline from the 1500s to 2009 is posted below the roof of the pavilion, explaining the history of the lake.

On the return trip, keep watch for birds in the trees. After a mile, you return to the end of the boardwalk and the beginning of the **Green Trail.** Turn left. Passing an outdoor classroom, the trail enters a picnic grove under the oaks. One live oak is the granddaddy of them all, tempting tree climbers with its low branches. The trail makes a sharp right to follow the fence line. Beyond the fence, and unmistakable, are creatures you normally don't see roaming around Central Florida: ibex, a herd of antelope, and an emu that came right up to the fence. There are benches and even a gazebo with a porch swing where you can sit and watch the animals as they come to feeding stations within easy view. The Green Trail reaches an intersection after the gazebo. Continue straight along the fence line. The trail emerges at the parking area after 1.3 miles.

Turn left and walk uphill past the parking area to the nature center. Just beyond it you'll find a post tipped with orange, the start of the **Uplands Trail,** which begins amid interpreted native plants and turns to parallel the entrance road through the pine woods. Taking the left junction at a **Nature Trail** sign leads you to a large shelter at a walk-in entrance from the West Orange Trail. There are benches and a water fountain at this shelter, as well as interpretive information about Lake Apopka and the preserve.

Leaving the shelter, turn left. This long straightaway parallels the West Orange Trail beneath the deep shade of tall pines. You can see bicyclists whiz by above you. Beyond a bench, the trail levels off as a blue-blazed trail takes off downhill to the right. Stay on the upper trail. After 1.9 miles, you reach a bench facing the West Orange Trail.

The trail makes a sharp right to zigzag down the hillside and the tight stair-step of contour lines between the oaks. At the T-intersection, turn right, continuing downhill beneath oaks and young hickory trees. Reaching a four-way junction, follow the yellow markers to the left, where the trail descends to another bench. On the left is a depression marsh with some interesting cypress trees. At the next four-way junction, the trail emerges behind a subdivision's retention pond. A sign points to the right and says SINKHOLE. Take a peek and you'll find out that the marsh is *in* the sinkhole!

Return to the four-way junction at marker 10 and take a left to walk along the retention pond fence, following the **Red Trail.** Turn right to follow the **Red Trail** into the forest. Pass the next trail junction with the **Yellow** and **Orange Trails.** Continue straight to cross a bridge over a narrow fern-dotted waterway. Look upstream and you'll see a small floodplain forest in a depression fed by a seepage spring.

Once you've crossed the bridge, you reach a T-junction with a broad trail beneath the pines. Turn left to follow the **Blue Trail,** which

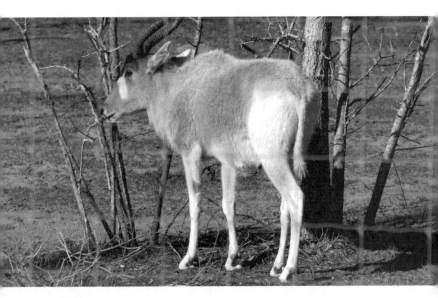

IBEX

leads right up to the back side of the nature center. If the gate isn't open to the back porch, continue around on the trail to the front of the nature center. If the center is open, stop and visit the displays, or just sit in a rocking chair and relax. Amble back to the parking lot to wrap up your 2.1-mile hike.

Nearby Attractions

Oakland adjoins Winter Garden, a historic community on Lake Apopka that is bisected by FL 438 and the popular West Orange Trail. Coffee shops and restaurants make the downtown area a delight to visit, and railroad buffs will find two fascinating museums: the Central Florida Railroad Museum (**cfcnrhs.org**) and the Winter Garden Heritage Museum (**wghf.org**).

Directions

From Florida's Turnpike, Exit 272 for Clermont/Winter Garden (FL 50), go east less than a mile to the first road on your left. There is no light or blinker, so it's tricky to cross traffic. There is a POST OFFICE sign here. Follow this road, Tubb Street, to its intersection with FL 438, Oakland Avenue. Turn left. Continue less than a mile, turning right at the sign for the nature preserve. Proceed through the front gate and follow the preserve road around to the parking area.

Tibet-Butler Preserve

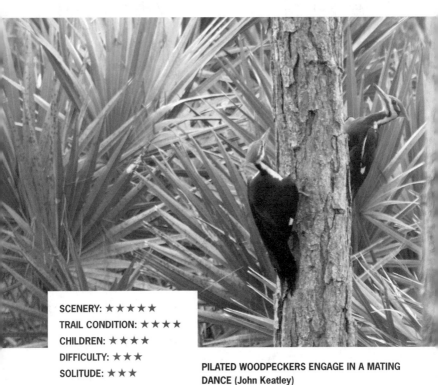

SCENERY: ★ ★ ★ ★ ★
TRAIL CONDITION: ★ ★ ★ ★
CHILDREN: ★ ★ ★ ★
DIFFICULTY: ★ ★ ★
SOLITUDE: ★ ★ ★

PILATED WOODPECKERS ENGAGE IN A MATING DANCE (John Keatley)

GPS TRAILHEAD COORDINATES: N28° 26.572' W81° 32.518'

DISTANCE & CONFIGURATION: 3-mile loop

HIKING TIME: 2 hours

HIGHLIGHTS: Palmetto Passage, observation deck, birding

ACCESS: Free; open Wednesday–Sunday, 8 a.m.–6 p.m.

MAPS: USGS *Windermere*

FACILITIES: Restrooms, picnic area with sandbox

WHEELCHAIR ACCESS: Limited to environmental center

COMMENTS: Some of the trails within the preserve (particularly Screech Owl and Palmetto Passage) can flood. Use alternative routes when those trails are posted closed.

CONTACTS: Tibet-Butler Preserve (407) 876-6696; **apps.ocfl.net/dept/CEsrvcs/Parks /ParkDetails.asp?ParkID=39**

Overview

One of the finest family hikes near Walt Disney World, Tibet-Butler Preserve is an oasis of wild natural habitats entirely surrounded by subdivisions within earshot of the whistle of the steam train at the Magic Kingdom. Encompassing 438 acres of pine flatwoods, bayhead swamp, scrub, and a cypress-lined shoreline on Lake Tibet, it is a complex of interconnecting trails radiating from the Vera Carter Environmental Center, a place for the kids (and you) to learn about the native habitats of this region.

Route Details

Leaving the parking area, wander through the environmental center for a quick lesson on habitats and wildlife and to find out what's new along the trail system. On the opposite side of the building, stop and sign in at the trail register. Descend to Pine Circle and turn right, snaking through the narrow passage between the saw palmetto to the **Screech Owl Trail.** Turn left. The trail follows the edge of the swamp, which you can see off to the right as the landscape drops down through marsh ferns. At the boardwalk, turn right to walk the Fallen Log Crossing.

Crossing water-filled hollows, the boardwalk heads into a thicket of loblolly bay and pines, zigzagging until it deposits you on a narrow footpath into the pine flatwoods. Blueberries form a natural hedge along the trail as the footpath turns grassy. Passing a bench, you reach the junction with the Palmetto Passage after 0.5 mile. Continue straight ahead. The forest closes in on the trail. Reaching a rain shelter, the trail meets the junction for the Osprey Overlook. Straight ahead is the **Tarflower Loop.** Continue straight ahead to walk into the scrub forest. Sand live oaks cast puddles of shade, while rusty lyonia show off their crooked stems. The trail narrows tightly, the diminutive trees covered in lichens. You reach a bench and a fence at the edge of the preserve. Turn left to tunnel into the scrub forest. As the loop continues around, you face the tall pines again. The trail narrows and, after 1.2 miles, completes the loop. Turn right.

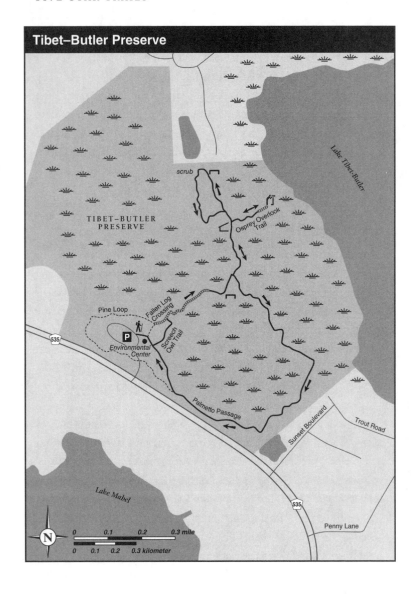

Tibet–Butler Preserve

Returning to the Osprey Overlook junction, turn left. Narrow and framed by saw palmetto, the trail enters a dense stand of pines. Rising up from the pine woods, a boardwalk guides you up over the marshy edge of Lake Tibet to an observation deck at 1.4 miles. The marsh bustles with bird life. Return along the Osprey Overlook to the junction. Turn left and walk back to the **Palmetto Passage.** This is the roughest, longest, and wildest of the trails in the preserve and frequently floods after heavy rains. All of this, however, makes it the most fun to hike. Turn left.

At the start, the trail is nicely groomed, with patches of deer moss and blueberries around the ever-present saw palmetto and loblolly bay. Then, the trail narrows and starts winding around beneath the low forest canopy, with a steady downhill trend toward the bayhead swamp. Since there are no blazes, just the faint impression of a path, it can be tricky to follow. Markers may be set in the ground at some of the points where you might otherwise lose your way. Crossing a log bridge, you can see where channels form as the bayhead spills over this rise and flows into the pine flatwoods. Logs and loose timbers serve as bog bridges in the low spots, although they may shift out of place when the water rises. Footing can be tricky. You cross what looks like a trail junction at 1.9 miles. Keep going straight ahead, reaching a patch of very old saw palmetto.

Winding through the woods, with lots of roots and some stumps underfoot, the trail continues under the low canopy of loblolly. After 2 miles, you must duck down in places to stay under the trees. Passing an arrow sign, the trail crosses a forest road and continues straight ahead. A patch of spongy lichens is squishy underfoot in a low spot. As the canopy opens, the trail gains elevation and you can see some houses off to the left and hear the slight buzz of traffic on the main road. Tacking through another part of the bayhead, the trail narrows tightly into a tunnel edged with loblolly bay. Tall slash pines and cypress trees grow along the swamp's edge. Gaining a little elevation, the footpath gets crunchy with the crackle of oak leaves underfoot. The trail is more deeply worn into the forest floor through the

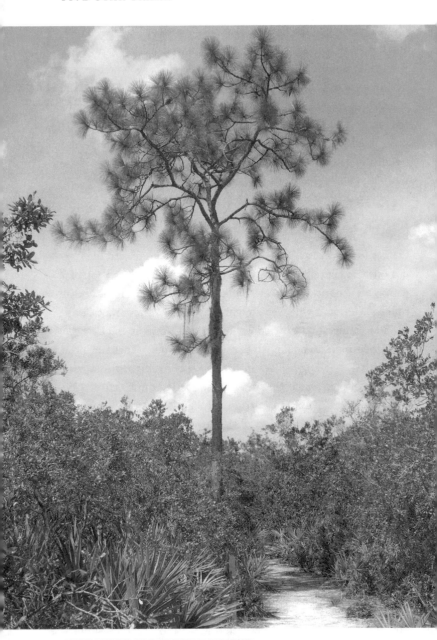

SCRUB FOREST AT TIBET-BUTLER PRESERVE

next section as it gets close to the road, twisting and turning before passing through a bog of ferns and sphagnum moss.

At 2.7 miles, the Palmetto Passage ends at a T-intersection with the Pine Circle. Since the Pine Circle loops the parking area and stays close to the road for a long segment, you may want to skip the full Pine Circle loop if you've completed the Palmetto Passage—consider it a higher, drier alternative to this trail. Turn right. Follow a short segment of the Pine Circle counterclockwise between the saw palmetto, passing the Screech Owl Trail on the right, to return to the Vera Carter Environmental Center. Sign out at the trail register and walk out to the parking area, completing a 3-mile hike.

Nearby Attractions

Tibet-Butler Preserve is just up the road from Walt Disney World's back (employee) gate, and only 5.5 miles from the Downtown Disney entrance to Walt Disney World: **disneyworld.com.**

Directions

Leaving I-4, Exit 68, drive north on Apopka/Vineland Road (FL 535). Pass the Downtown Disney entrance to Walt Disney World at the first light. Turn left at the second light onto County Road 535. Drive 5.3 miles to the park entrance on the right. The entrance road loops around to parking spots in front of the environmental center.

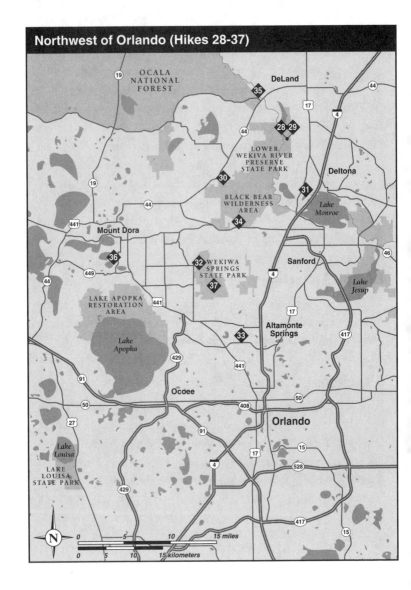

Northwest of Orlando (Hikes 28-37)

OCALA NATIONAL FOREST

DeLand

19

44

35

17

4

28 29

44

LOWER WEKIVA RIVER PRESERVE STATE PARK

Deltona

30

19

31

BLACK BEAR WILDERNESS AREA

Lake Monroe

441

44

Mount Dora

34

36

449

32 WEKIWA SPRINGS STATE PARK

Sanford

46

44

37

4

Lake Jesup

LAKE APOPKA RESTORATION AREA

441

Altamonte Springs

17

417

Lake Apopka

33

91

429

441

Ocoee

50

408

50

27

91

Orlando

15

Lake Louisa

LAKE LOUISA STATE PARK

4

17

528

429

417

15

N

0   5   10   15 miles

0   5   10   15 kilometers

Northwest

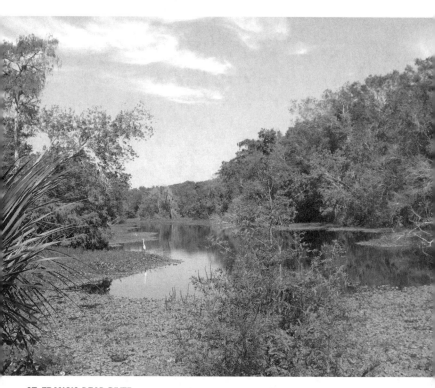

ST. FRANCIS DEAD RIVER

Blue Spring State Park: Blue Spring Trail

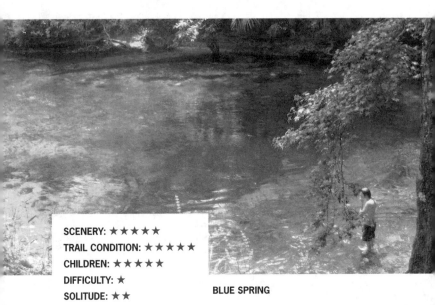

SCENERY: ★ ★ ★ ★ ★

TRAIL CONDITION: ★ ★ ★ ★ ★

CHILDREN: ★ ★ ★ ★ ★

DIFFICULTY: ★

SOLITUDE: ★ ★

BLUE SPRING

GPS TRAILHEAD COORDINATES: N28° 56.542' W81° 20.465'

DISTANCE & CONFIGURATION: 1.5-mile out-and-back

HIKING TIME: 1 hour

HIGHLIGHTS: Views of Blue Spring Run, manatee sightings

ACCESS: $4 individual entrance fee, $6 per carload; open daily, 8 a.m.–sunset

MAPS: USGS *Orange City*

FACILITIES: Restrooms, picnic area, playground, campground, cabins, camp store, gift shop, swimming area, canoe and kayak rentals, guided ecotours

WHEELCHAIR ACCESS: Entirely wheelchair-accessible

COMMENTS: Park closes its gates when parking capacity is reached, which can happen early on winter weekends. All water-based activities in Blue Spring Run (swimming, paddling, scuba) are closed during manatee season. However, paddlers can still launch into the St. Johns River and explore other nearby waterways.

CONTACTS: Blue Spring State Park (386) 775-3663; **floridastateparks.org/bluespring**

Overview

If you've never seen manatees by the dozens, let alone a hundred or more, there's no better place in Florida to watch these gentle giants drift past than near DeLand, along the boardwalk at Blue Spring State Park, paralleling the length of Blue Spring Run to the St. Johns River. This short, easy trail offers plenty of viewing platforms where you can stand and stare at the mystically beautiful movement of these massive mammals through crystalline waters. This clear spring has become a mecca for a rebounding manatee population over the past three decades, with their winter gathering growing exponentially each year.

Route Details

Start your walk with a meander past the restrooms and picnic pavilions to the St. Johns River landing from the lower parking area. It's where Blue Spring Run flows into the St. Johns River, and the landing offers a panorama of the river bend, the spring run mouth, and "The Lagoon." Looping around the lagoon is the Pine Island Trail (Hike 29, page 189). Wading birds frequent the shorelines, and you'll see coots and gallinules in the river shallows. Watch the mouth of the spring for manatee activity. The manatees drift past most frequently after dawn and before dusk. They will be moving from the spring run, where their steady diet of aquatic plants is severely limited, to the open river and its many side channels to feed on vegetation.

Leaving the landing, turn left and walk past the ticket booth for the river tour uphill along the broad boardwalk. A notable landmark at the top of the hill is the Thursby House, built in 1872. It was one of the first plantation homes along the St. Johns River. Its steamboat landing encouraged the growth of Orange City, which was known back then for its citrus that was shipped from the landing. Decorated with period furnishings, the plantation house is open for tours.

As you continue along the boardwalk, notice how the hills become much more pronounced the closer you get to the spring. Excavations in the area have uncovered pottery shards and tools made from seashells

Blue Spring State Park: Blue Spring Trail

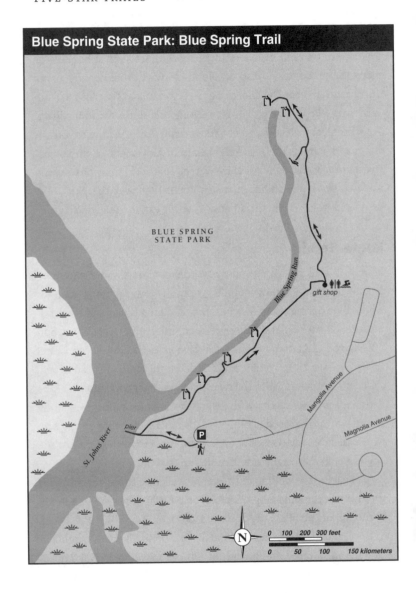

in middens along the sides of the spring run, making this a significant archaeological site as well as a historical site and wildlife sanctuary. You'll pass a canoe launch on the left, and soon after, encounter the first of three large observation decks. If it seems too crowded, just move along and try the next one—you'll be returning this way anyway.

Branches arc out across the water from the dense forest of live oaks on the far side of the spring run, creating perfect perches for cormorants that cluster close together as they dry their wings. Look straight down. The water is so clear that the fish seem to float in air. Long, large alligator gar cruise past. But you're here, of course, for the manatees. Usually, the best way to spot a manatee is to look for the spring boil–like disturbance of the water's surface as they rise. But in Blue Spring Run, the water is so clear that all you have to do is look carefully for their telltale bulk. They may be scratching their backs against fallen logs, cruising past with calves, or chomping on fallen vegetation. Stand here for a while, and you're sure to spot one, as their sheer numbers practically guarantee it. Recent counts have hovered close to 200 in the spring run each winter.

Park personnel have worked to optimize the manatee viewing experience along this walk. Low vegetation has been cleared so that the boardwalk provides a continuous view of the spring run as you ascend upstream. The boardwalk narrows past the Thursby House, providing a shady corridor in the woods while you spy on the manatees from high above. Broad spots and observation decks offer a variety of views of the animals. In the winter, as the water temperature in the St. Johns River and its tributaries drops below 68°F, manatees crowd into Blue Spring Run to warm up in the constant 72°F water, essential for their survival. Each adult manatee can weigh more than a ton. At this time of year, you'll see a lot of mothers and calves cruising together through the shallows. It's worth visiting the swimming area (closed this time of year) for the potential of an up-close look as manatees swim under the platform resting on the run.

The boardwalk continues through a beehive of activity at the park store and main picnic area, where there are restrooms. It quiets down and narrows again past the building and is signposted here as the **Blue Spring Trail.** It's here that the pronounced topography gets very interesting, the boardwalk lifted high above side channels of the run between ancient middens swaddled in cabbage palms and live oaks. A lengthy side boardwalk leads down to the water and is the launch point for divers and swimmers to explore the headspring during the summer season. It offers yet another place to see manatees up close. As the trail reaches the headspring, it enters a large pavilion with interpretive information about how the aquifer works and how deep into the earth this spring has been mapped. The boardwalk swings around to offer another perspective, this one straight down Blue Spring Run, and stops at this high point after 0.7 mile. Savor the view before you turn around and walk back down the boardwalk to the St. Johns River and the parking area, pausing again at the various overlooks to be caught up in the magic of watching manatees move through the crystalline waters.

Nearby Attractions

The Pine Island Trail (Hike 29, page 189) starts from the far end of the same parking area. Departing from the landing at the floating dock near the parking area, St. Johns River Cruises offers two-hour tours on a smooth-riding, quiet pontoon boat. Fully wheelchair-accessible, these narrated nature tours take you up the St. Johns River toward Hontoon Island and into some of the side channels, such as the Snake River, for birding and wildlife encounters: **sjrivercruises.com.**

Directions

Take I-4 east from Orlando to Exit 114. Head northeast on FL 472 for 3.5 miles to US 17/92 south. Take US 17/92 south toward Orange City for 1.5 miles. Turn right on West French Street. A large overhead state park sign calls your attention to the turn. The paved road ends after several miles. The park entrance is on the left. After you pay your fee, take the left fork to drive to the lower parking area.

29 # Blue Spring State Park: Pine Island Trail

SCENERY: ★ ★ ★ ★
TRAIL CONDITION: ★ ★ ★ ★
CHILDREN: ★ ★
DIFFICULTY: ★ ★ ★ ★
SOLITUDE: ★ ★ ★

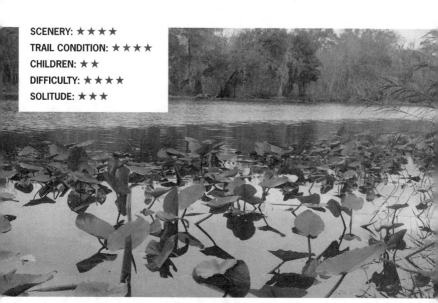

ST. JOHNS RIVER AT THE END OF THE PINE ISLAND TRAIL

GPS TRAILHEAD COORDINATES: N28° 56.551' W81° 20.402'

DISTANCE & CONFIGURATION: 7.3-mile out-and-back

HIKING TIME: 4.5 hours

HIGHLIGHTS: Dense palm and oak hammocks, cypress swamps, scrub-jay sightings, St. Johns River shoreline

ACCESS: $4 individual entrance fee, $6 per carload; open daily, 8 a.m.–sunset

MAPS: USGS *Orange City*

FACILITIES: Restrooms, picnic area, playground, campground, cabins, camp store, gift shop, swimming area, canoe and kayak rentals, guided ecotours

WHEELCHAIR ACCESS: None

COMMENTS: The trail is signposted with an incorrect mileage (4.5 miles each way) near the trailhead. More than 2 miles are in full sun; use sun protection. Mosquito repellent is also advised.

CONTACTS: Blue Spring State Park (386) 775-3663; **floridastateparks.org/bluespring**

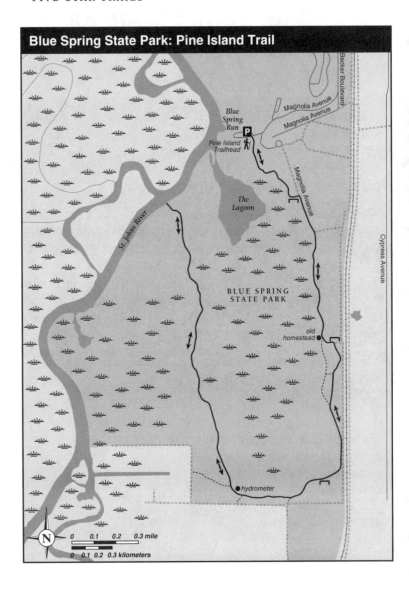

Blue Spring State Park: Pine Island Trail

Overview

Starting near the exit of the lower parking area, the Pine Island Trail at Blue Spring State Park is lesser known and lesser used than its popular counterpart, the Blue Spring Trail (and boardwalk) along Blue Spring Run. It might be the distance—7.3 miles round-trip— or the terrain. The going isn't easy at first, but it's worth pushing through the scrub habitats, where you might see Florida scrub-jays, to get to the spectacular pine, oak, and palm forests en route to the St. Johns River.

Route Details

The **Pine Island Trail** starts near the exit of the lower parking loop. A kiosk at the trailhead contains a rough map of the trail. It's an out-and-back walk to the St. Johns River around a very large lagoon, transitioning between bone-dry and soggy habitats as it makes a large horseshoe curve. Passing the warning sign (where the mileage is incorrect), the hike starts out in a hardwood hammock with a smattering of southern magnolias among the oaks and is marked, occasionally, with a bootprint symbol on a post. To the right, not far off, is the floodplain forest that edges the lagoon. Gaining some elevation, the trail passes under older loblolly pines, some with signs of turpentine tapping, and scattered American holly.

The understory becomes a thicket on the left as the trail transitions into scrub under the oak trees, with towering rusty lyonia, some rising to tree size, overhead. A line of light to the left through the trees belies how close you are drawing to the open scrub, which is in the process of being restored to ideal Florida scrub-jay habitat. At 0.4 mile you reach a bench and a T-intersection with a forest road. Power lines rise in the distance beyond a flat, mostly featureless restoration area. Turn right. Walking along the edge of this restoration area, which is awaiting new growth, the views aren't especially pretty. You pass a road leading off to the left to a line of trees in the distance. The trail slips between the scrub and a mixed oak and pine forest to the right; a line of cabbage palms in the distance on the right marks the edge of the lagoon.

There is no shade, and it gets hot quickly. Passing milepost 1, the trail jogs back and forth a little. Listen closely and you may hear the "shreep" of a scrub-jay in the distance. Around the next bend are the remains of a homestead, complete with foundation and cistern. A spill of fossilized snail shells across the ground lends a clue that the home probably sat atop fill taken from an ancient Timucuan midden. The trail sweeps upward to the left, becoming deep, soft sand underfoot as it leaves the tree line at a fork. At the top of the hill, it passes a bench as it curves to the right and into the heart of the scrub. After you pass a road on the right, the elevation drops. The sand transitions to a firmer footpath underfoot, a grassy road along the pond pines. By 1.6 miles, the trail draws close to the park boundary fence and the power line briefly before swinging away from the fence and into the pond pine forest in a slow descent.

Reaching a bench at 1.8 miles, you're now firmly into denser forest and will remain in a series of forests through the end of the trail. That difficult section of open scrub is behind you until the return trip. Unfortunately, many people turn back before this point, not realizing the "truly worth hiking" part of this trail is past this rough section. Pines and oaks rise well overhead, denser on the south side of the trail. You feel a distinct drop in air temperature as the trail drops down into a floodplain between two small stretches of oak scrub. Past a spur to the fence line on the left, the trail keeps dropping in elevation, passing a massive pine tree on the right. At 2 miles you dip into a beautiful cypress swamp with a wondrous interplay of floodplain plants. If you have to wade through this swamp and the wading is more than ankle-deep, the trail will be impassable from flooding farther on. Except for those scrub uplands, the entire Pine Island Trail is easily affected by the rise and fall of the St. Johns River, with the lagoon creeping beyond its marshes and into the woods. If this section of trail is dry, you should have easy going the rest of the way.

As you rise out of the floodplain, the trail is flanked with massive live oaks, their gnarled limbs covered in bromeliads and resurrection ferns. You pass a back gate to the park on the left. The trail climbs upward into a patch of scrubby flatwoods with only a smattering of shade. Past a hydrology station at 2.5 miles, the trail curves to the left into the deep shade of a lush hammock of palms, pines, and large live oaks. While the trail continues to descend, more oaks and pines fill the forest, and you feel a cool breeze from the St. Johns River. Saw palmetto crowds closely as the trail narrows, and pinecones spill across the rooty footpath. Passing a bootprint marker and a mileage marker at 3 miles, you continue the descent under the limbs of ancient oaks. As the trail snakes downhill, you follow its curves through another palm hammock in the floodplain. At a low spot in the trail, the lagoon can spill over and swamp the trail; there are old footbridges, strewn by floodwaters, in the high grasses to the right. You may have to wade this short section, except in the driest of seasons.

Rising out of the floodplain into a palm hammock where the outspread limbs of live oaks form horizontal counterpoints to the verticals of the palm trunks, the trail enters its final and most beautiful section. This slight ridge above the St. Johns River is home to an ancient forest that envelops the trail in deep shade from its high canopy. The trail narrows more, squeezed by saw palmetto through a short stretch of pines. You can see a ribbon of sky up ahead through the trees. Descending back into the hammock, you pass an unusable privy (the primitive campsites here were washed away and abandoned after the hurricanes of 2004), and the trail narrows more tightly. Follow it as it slips between the trees, past the old markers for the campsites, and makes a sharp left before it pops out on the banks on the St. Johns River after 3.6 miles, just beyond a "Mile 4" sign. A sweeping view of the river is before you; sparkling mussel shells and colorful wildflowers line the shores.

Since this is an out-and-back hike, you must retrace your steps. Savor the slow ascent beneath the deeply shaded hammocks. You'll feel the elevation gain by the time you rise out of the cypress swamp and keep walking uphill into the oaks and pines at 5.5 miles. Pausing at the bench in the woods, keep hydrated to gather your strength for that short but energy-sapping push across the soft sand of the open scrub on the way out. Don't miss that all-important turn at the bench at 6.9 miles to reenter the last stretch of forest, that final shady portion en route to the trailhead. You complete the hike after 7.3 miles.

Nearby Attractions

The Blue Spring Trail (Hike 28, page 184) starts at the other end of the parking area. Departing from the landing at the floating dock, St. Johns River Cruises offers two-hour tours on a smooth-riding, quiet pontoon boat. Fully wheelchair-accessible, these narrated nature tours take you up the St. Johns River toward Hontoon Island and into some of the side channels, such as the Snake River, for birding and wildlife encounters: **sjrivercruises.com.**

Directions

Take I-4 east from Orlando to Exit 114. Head northeast on FL 472 for 3.5 miles to US 17/92 south. Take US 17/92 south toward Orange City for 1.5 miles. Turn right on West French Street. A large overhead state park sign calls your attention to the turn. The paved road ends after several miles. The park entrance is on the left. After you pay your fee, take the left fork to drive to the lower parking area.

Florida Trail: Seminole State Forest

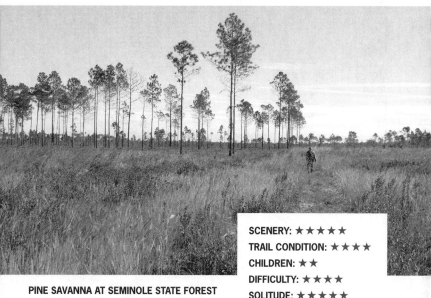

SCENERY: ★ ★ ★ ★ ★
TRAIL CONDITION: ★ ★ ★ ★
CHILDREN: ★ ★
DIFFICULTY: ★ ★ ★ ★
SOLITUDE: ★ ★ ★ ★ ★

PINE SAVANNA AT SEMINOLE STATE FOREST

GPS TRAILHEAD COORDINATES:

Cassia Trailhead: N28° 53.399' W81° 27.695'

Bear Pond Trailhead: N28° 49.152' W81° 25.683'

DISTANCE & CONFIGURATION: 7.6-mile one-way, with shuttle

HIKING TIME: 4 hours

HIGHLIGHTS: Blackwater Creek, Shark Tooth Spring, open prairie

ACCESS: $2 per person; open 24/7

MAPS: USGS *Pine Lakes* and *Sanford SW*

FACILITIES: Privies at both trailheads, picnic pavilion at Bear Pond Trailhead, picnic table at Blackwater Creek, trailside benches in several spots, trail shelter

WHEELCHAIR ACCESS: None

COMMENTS: Excellent habitat for Florida black bear and Florida scrub-jay.

CONTACTS: Florida Forest Service, Leesburg Forestry Station (352) 360-6675 or (352) 360-6677; **floridaforestservice.com/state_forests**

Florida Trail: Seminole State Forest

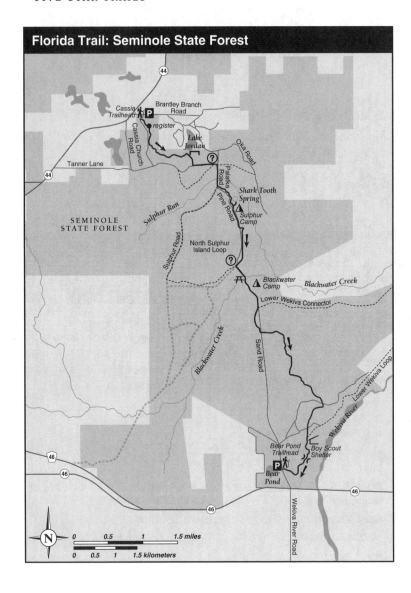

Overview

Heading south along a segment of the statewide Florida Trail, this hike through Seminole State Forest showcases vast, open prairies that you'd never imagine existed on such a grand scale so close to an urban area. Yet it's not a one-note trail. Rugged hills, colorful swamp forests, palm hammocks dense with leafy cabbage palms, and an abundance of wildlife add to the experience. With access to the Shark Tooth Spring, which spits out fossilized sharks' teeth, and to a picnic table along scenic Blackwater Creek, it's a hike where you'll want to take the time for a little trailside exploration.

Route Details

To hike the Florida Trail through Seminole State Forest, you'll need to pre-arrange a shuttle back to your car at the Cassia Trailhead or hike with a friend, leaving one car at the end point at the Bear Pond Trailhead (see "Directions" on page 200) before you start off from the Cassia Trailhead.

From the Cassia Trailhead, the orange-blazed Florida Trail sweeps through a frame of live oaks to enter the woods. After rounding a large sinkhole on the left, you'll find a trail register and map in this forest of pines and oaks. From the top of a small hill, you will see a forest road off to the right. Longleaf pines tower overhead near a large, well-established sinkhole. After a corridor of saw palmetto, the trail emerges into an open area along a large, wet prairie where sandhill cranes gather. Upon leaving the prairie, the footpath passes between two fence posts to enter a sand pine scrub forest with bright-white sand underfoot, crossing a sand road at 1 mile. An opening on the left provides a bench with a sweeping view of Boggy Creek Lake.

Emerging onto a forest road, the trail turns left. Watch for blazing, as many equestrian trails intersect here. An orange blaze is on the kiosk at 1.6 miles. Turn right and walk down Palatka Road. Canopied, shady, almost junglelike, the forest envelops you, and the air temperature drops. Cypresses outline a stream in the distance. Crossing several culverts, the road rises to an intersection with Pine Road. It's easy to lose the trail here if you're not alert. The orange blazes do not follow the roads but turn downhill to the left into the tall underbrush. You don't see a confirmation blaze until you step past the first saw palmetto and down. The trail clings to a hill, winding its way downhill and back up at a sharp angle. Be cautious of roots underfoot.

Where the trail reaches a T-intersection at 2.4 miles, turn left down the spur trail to Shark Tooth Spring. This trail narrows and narrows until you expect a troll to pop out at the bridge and demand coins for passage. Pouring out of a hole in the hill, the crystalline stream flows beneath the palms. Stick your hand in the water and stir up the sand. You'll find small, black fossilized sharks' teeth that the spring perpetually spits out of the earth.

Return back up the spur trail and pass the incoming trail on the right, ending up in a large, grassy campsite with a fire ring and picnic table. Pass through the posts on the far side and reach a T-intersection with a forest road. Blue blazes to the right mark the Sulphur Island Loop, a Trailwalker Trail within Seminole State Forest. Turn left to follow the orange blazes. The trail leaves the road to the right almost immediately. It parallels the road but in the beauty of the sand pine scrub, the forest floor fluffy with seafoam-colored deer moss.

Watch for a sharp right at the next T-intersection that leads down an old tramway built by loggers to remove the prize giants of this forest a century or more ago. The tramway yields to a very tight tunnel of saw palmetto to push though. Cross a trail with the forest road off to your right. The next forest road crossing is at 3.1 miles. Past a dry prairie pond, the trail gets into deeper shade.

Emerging at an intersection of roads with a trail kiosk, turn left. The orange blazes lead down Sand Road. By 3.5 miles, you reach the picnic tables that overlook a lazy bend on picturesque Blackwater Creek, which is as broad as most Florida rivers. It drains Lake Norris through Seminole State Forest to reach the Wekiva River. Continue across the bridge and watch for blazes. At 3.7 miles, you pass a blue-blazed trail to the left that connects to the upper end of the Lower

Wekiva Loop (Hike 34, page 217). Continue along the road, looking for a blaze post and FLORIDA TRAIL sign to lead you back into the woods. The trail narrows down from a broad swath to a rough-mown path, and you cross a small bridge over an ephemeral wetland. To the east, the landscape rolls off to the horizon, an expansive view above the saw palmetto.

At 4.5 miles, you cross Main Grade Road to be immersed in this spectacular landscape. Tall grasses wave in the breeze. If you're here for an out-and-back hike, use this spot as your turnaround point so you sample the best of the landscapes along the trail for a 9-mile out-and-back hike.

While the trail is a straightaway for some time, it jogs around a wet prairie briefly, crossing a few bog bridges. The grasslands just go on and on, and all you can do is marvel at their vastness in this setting. Trail junctions with unmarked trails can be confusing, but keep watching for the next orange blaze. Reaching a desert island in this sea of prairie—bright-white sands from ancient seas—the footpath enters a scrub forest where the Florida scrub-jay reigns. Bright blue, very vocal, and larger than a robin, these birds are only found in Florida and only in remnants of these ancient habitats.

Crossing a broad sand road, the trail winds into scrubby flatwoods, a damp habitat where minuscule sundew plants rise from the footpath in glistening patches of red. As you gain elevation, you cross the next sand road into a slightly rolling landscape of ancient dunes and fluffy young sand pines, passing an interpretive sign about the Florida scrub-jay at 6.5 miles. At the end of a corridor of pines you'll find the next trail register box and the intersection with the Lower Wekiva Loop (Hike 34, page 217). Both trails follow the same route from here to their terminus at the Bear Pond Trailhead.

Turning left at the T-intersection, you reach the Boy Scout shelter, a large three-sided camping area. Continue through the clearing and along a broad, grassy corridor. The footpath eases right and becomes a narrow track, narrowing more tightly as you enter the first shady forest you've encountered in nearly 4 miles of hiking. The trail crosses a bridge at 7.1 miles, with a directional post noting 0.5 MILES TO ENTRANCE. After a ramble beneath tall pines, you pass an old hand-lettered sign with trail mileages just before reaching Bear Pond Trailhead, the southern terminus of the hike.

Nearby Attractions

Seminole State Forest touches several other public lands within the Wekiva River Basin with hiking trails that are not covered by this book, including Lower Wekiva River Preserve State Park and Rock Springs Run Reserve State Park, both accessible from FL 46: **floridastateparks .org.** Just east of the Bear Pond Trailhead entrance, Wekiva Falls RV Resort, a KOA Campground, offers waterslides, canoeing, and kayaking: **wekivafallsresort.com.**

Directions

To Bear Pond Trailhead (south end): From I-4, Exit 101C at Sanford, take FL 46 west for 5.2 miles. After you cross the Wekiva River, look for the entrance to Seminole State Forest on the right. Continue for 1 mile along the forest road—stopping at the self-service kiosk to pay the day-use fee—to park on the left.

To Cassia Trailhead (north end): Continue west on FL 46 from the Seminole State Forest entrance for 2.2 miles to the traffic light with FL 46A. Drive north 5.6 miles to the traffic light with FL 44. Turn right and drive 5.1 miles east on FL 44 to Brantley Branch Road on the right. Turn right. The Cassia Trailhead will be on your right.

Gemini Springs Park

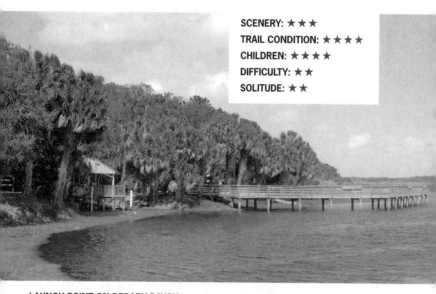

SCENERY: ★ ★ ★
TRAIL CONDITION: ★ ★ ★ ★
CHILDREN: ★ ★ ★ ★
DIFFICULTY: ★ ★
SOLITUDE: ★ ★

LAUNCH POINT ON DEBARY BAYOU

GPS TRAILHEAD COORDINATES: N28° 51.845' W81° 18.566'

DISTANCE & CONFIGURATION: 2.2-mile loop

HIKING TIME: 1.5 hours

HIGHLIGHTS: Gemini Springs, views of the bayou, ancient oaks, archaeological sites

ACCESS: Free; open daily, sunrise–sunset

MAPS: USGS *Sanford*

FACILITIES: Playground, restrooms, picnic tables and grills, picnic pavilions, paved bicycle trail, dog park, kayak and canoe rentals, fishing pier, canoe launch, group campsite

WHEELCHAIR ACCESS: Yes, using the paved trails

COMMENTS: The park is a trailhead for the Spring-to-Spring Trail, a bicycle path that connects to Green Spring Park (Hike 3, page 38). Leashed pets permitted.

CONTACTS: Volusia County Government Parks, Recreation and Culture (386) 736-5953; **volusia.org/parks/gemini.htm**

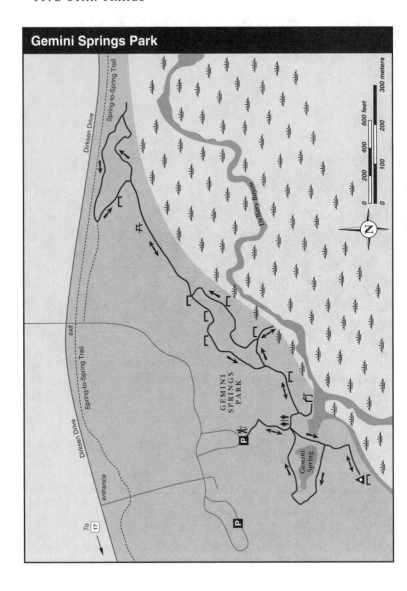

Gemini Springs Park

Overview

More than 150 years ago, this forest along the marshes of the St. Johns River was cleared for farming, becoming the Padgett homestead on the outskirts of busy Enterprise. It later operated as a cattle ranch for the Gray family, who built the dam and reservoir, the spring house, and arched bridges. In 1994, the land became a 210-acre preserve protecting its namesake springs and archaeological sites. With its mix of gentle woodland paths and paved trails, playgrounds, picnic area, paddling trail, and dog park, Gemini Springs Park is a popular local getaway for outdoor recreation just off I-4.

Route Details

Walk down the path from the parking area past the restrooms, and turn left. Wander down to the boardwalk deck at the canoe-rental area, as it offers a sweeping view of DeBary Bayou, part of the St. Johns River. Just past the canoe launch, the concrete path yields to a natural surface trail into an oak hammock, where Spanish moss thickly drapes the ancient live oaks. Near a bench, interpretive signs talk about the habitat and the trees you'll see in this shady hammock. The air is scented with orange blossoms; citrus trees grow beneath the ancient oaks, reminders of the homesteading era.

At the trail junction, turn right. A blue hiker marker confirms the route. There is a small clearing with a bench and information about the historic DeBary Estate, established in the 1870s by wine merchant Frederick deBary as a hunting estate. Turn right for a short walk out to the bayou's edge. Returning to the bench, continue straight ahead down the grassy path beneath the oaks and palms. Passing another bench, a trail goes off to the left. Continue straight. You can hear the buzz of the interstate in the distance. On the left, the oak hammock yields to a floodplain forest with water oaks, red maples, and bald cypress along the bayou's fringe. At 0.6 mile there is a bench at a junction of trails adjoining mounds of grapevine beneath a large longleaf pine. Turn right.

The trail becomes a grassy path under tall slash pines and fragrant elderberry. The forest to the right is thick with ferns, among them netted chain, cinnamon, and royal ferns. Reaching the next junction, continue straight ahead. A picnic table hides between the trees at this fork. Reaching a T-intersection, jog to the right to continue down this outer trail. Virginia willows appear through gaps in the forest, outlining the rim of the bayou. As the trail curves to the right, young cedars create a grove. At the next fork in the trail, turn left to begin back around the loop. Dirksen Drive is not far through the woods, and you can hear a little traffic from it. The oaks are younger here, a second-growth forest with water oaks and sweetgum. The park boundary fence is nearby, with the Spring-to-Spring Trail— a paved bicycle route to Green Spring Park (Hike 3, page 38).

Passing a primeval-looking patch of cinnamon ferns, you come to a T-intersection. Keep right to stay on the outer loop, passing a cross trail that heads back toward the picnic table. The trees are much shorter here, almost scrubby, but provide shade for the footpath. At the next junction, there are tall pines among the oaks. Turn left amid a tangle of blackberry bushes covered in grapevines. At 1 mile, there is a bench with a trail off to the left. Continue straight. At the next T-intersection, turn right, and then right again. You pass the picnic table, returning along the trail closest to the bayou. When you reach the four-way intersection with the bench, go straight ahead.

Walking beneath the ancient live oaks again, you come up to the next junction with a bench. Look off to the left and you can see the open area near the bayou. Continue straight. The trail winds through the forest, dense with grapevines in the understory. A blocked-off trail to the right leads to the picnic area near the restrooms. Returning to the part of the forest where the citrus trees thrive under the tall canopy of oaks, the trail reaches a three-way junction. Continue straight, returning to the sidewalk again at 1.5 miles. Turn left to follow the concrete path across the dam for panoramic views of the palm-lined bayou shore, the bayou itself, and the spring pool behind the reservoir.

On the far side of the waterway, more paved paths lead through the forest. It's a nice diversion to walk down to the right and to the edge of the bayou for more sweeping views. Return to the main path, and circle the spring pool. Swimming is not allowed here, but waterfowl, especially egrets and herons, find the clear waters inviting.

The paved path reaches a small bridge at the north end of the reservoir, where a waterway flows in. Loop around to start walking down the other side, where you'll find a small overlook over one of the springs. Together, the cluster of springs pours up to 6.5 million gallons of fresh water into the St. Johns River each day. Skirt around the spring house and cross another bridge before this path brings you back around to the start of the nature trail. Turn left to exit to the parking area, completing a 2.2-mile walk.

Nearby Attractions

Just up the street is DeBary Hall, the manor house of the 1870s estate that once encompassed a portion of this park. Guided historical tours and ecoadventures are offered: **debaryhall.com.**

Directions

From I-4, Exit 108, go west on Dirksen Drive for 1.6 miles to the park entrance. Turn left and enter the park road. Where the park road splits, keep left and make the first right to head down to the canoe-launch area.

32 Kelly Park

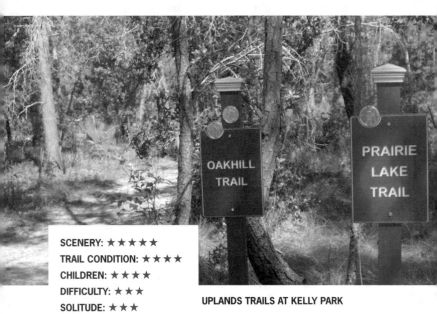

SCENERY: ★ ★ ★ ★ ★
TRAIL CONDITION: ★ ★ ★ ★
CHILDREN: ★ ★ ★ ★
DIFFICULTY: ★ ★
SOLITUDE: ★ ★

UPLANDS TRAILS AT KELLY PARK

GPS TRAILHEAD COORDINATES: N28° 45.437' W81° 30.031'

DISTANCE & CONFIGURATION: 4-mile loop and balloon

HIKING TIME: 2 hours

HIGHLIGHTS: Rock Springs Run, sinkholes and springs, wildlife-watching

ACCESS: $3–$5 per vehicle; open daily 8 a.m.–8 p.m. in summer, 8 a.m.–6 p.m. in winter

MAPS: USGS *Sanford SW* and *Pine Lakes*

FACILITIES: Restrooms, picnic pavilions, playground, campground, swimming area, tubing run, food concession (summer months), bathhouse, lockers

WHEELCHAIR ACCESS: Limited to sidewalks and boardwalks near the spring run

COMMENTS: As a popular swimming hole, Kelly Park gets extremely crowded on summer days. The gates are closed once the parking area reaches capacity. Campers, however, can come and go freely.

CONTACTS: Kelly Park (407) 889-4179; **apps.ocfl.net/dept/CEsrvcs/Parks/ParkDetails .asp?ParkID=22**

Overview

One of the region's oldest public parks, Kelly Park dates back to 1927, when it was given to the people of Apopka by Dr. Howard Atwood Kelly, one of the founders of Johns Hopkins University. Protecting the source of Rock Springs Run, a cavern in a very tropical setting, the park features one of the prettiest tubing runs in Florida. The trail system includes loops both inside and outside the park gates, providing scenic views of the crystalline waterway, as well as an up-close look at karst topography, with sinkholes and springs along the route.

Route Details

Start your hike by walking from the parking area to the concession stand. Walk through it to your first view of the swimming area and Rock Springs Run from a platform on the hill. The boardwalk along the run heads uphill and is easy to follow; tens of thousands of visitors walk this each year as they carry tubes up to the source of the run for a cool ride downstream. The boardwalk zigzags downhill to meander along the waterway and a scene that seems almost dreamlike: stretches of rock rimmed with ferns past which turquoise-tinted waters flow above sparkling sands. The bridge crosses in front of Rock Springs, a cavern of significant size from which the waterway emerges, pushing 26,000 gallons of pure spring water past you each minute. With children splashing and snorkelers in the 68-degree outflow, it's quite the sight.

After crossing the bridge, walk uphill, away from the spring and the lifeguard's chair. It's here, after 0.25 mile, you find your first sign for the trail system, **Kelly Loop Trail.** Make a right at the fork. At the next intersection, go straight across to the next sign. Look for yellow blazes to confirm the route. The trail is a broad path through the upland hammock. There is obvious topography to the trail as you climb away from the spring basin, passing a bench. One of the joys of this hike is the ups and downs created by the spring basin and upland sinkholes.

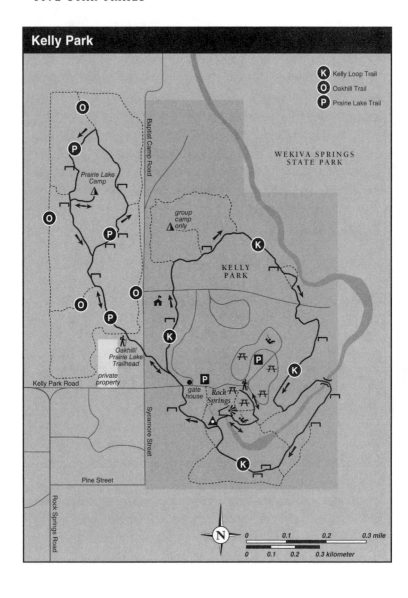

Kelly Park

K Kelly Loop Trail
O Oakhill Trail
P Prairie Lake Trail

WEKIVA SPRINGS
STATE PARK

KELLY
PARK

group
camp
only

Prairie Lake
Camp

Baptist Camp Road

Oakhill/
Prairie Lake
Trailhead

private
property

Kelly Park Road

gate
house

Rock
Springs

Sycamore Street

Pine Street

Rock Springs Road

N

0   0.1   0.2   0.3 mile

0   0.1   0.2   0.3 kilometer

Cross the park road within sight of the entrance station. The trail continues as a bark-chip path in the median toward the front entrance. Leave this path at the first green post to walk out the park gate and across the road to the fire station. Cross the open area to the right of the firehouse to reach a gap in the fence at the far fence line. This secondary trail system, consisting of the **Oakhill Trail** and **Prairie Lake Trail,** offers a different perspective on the uplands around the spring basin. Start down the shaded forest road, which leads you into the loop-trail system using both red and blue blazes. At the fork, stay right to follow the red blazes of the **Prairie Lake Trail.** Keep right at the next fork. The trail passes a bench flanked by saw palmettos and curves around a deep, well-established sinkhole. Stay left at the next fork, following the blue blazes.

The trail emerges from the woods and skirts what was once the shoreline of Prairie Lake at 1 mile. One of the sad realities of the karst landscape is that springs can dry up. Sometimes it happens due to natural causes, such as a blockage underground, but more often it's due to overwithdrawal from the aquifer by surrounding wells. It has been several decades since Prairie Lake was nourished by its springs. The prairie is rimmed by scrub forest, and you pass a bench overlooking this open area before the trail sweeps back into the shade afforded by the oaks, which form a tightly knit low canopy.

Emerging into the sandhills, the trail continues beneath young turkey oaks. At the triple junction of trails, you're at the top of the loop of the two intertwined trails. The Oakhill Trail continues to the north. Turn left to stay on the Prairie Lake Trail. The habitat transitions into hardwood forest. An arm of the prairie reaches into the woods, and the trail is slightly elevated as if it were on a causeway. Cabbage palms grow along the prairie rim, which the trail follows. At the next junction, turn right, following the red arrows. Another connector trail comes in from the left, leading to Prairie Lake Camp, an open spot for primitive camping. The footpath returns to the sandhill habitat, with tall slash pines and oaks shading the trail. When you reach the next trail junction, you've completed the big loop. Continue ahead on the broad forest road to the gap in the fence, exiting this trail system at 1.9 miles. Walk around the fire station and cross the road.

Once you're back inside the park gates, head for the trees on the left. A well-beaten path leads under the pines to rejoin the **Kelly Loop Trail** at an intersection just before the campground road. Turn left. The trail swoops down sharply into a sinkhole. Outlined by boards, the footpath rounds a series of sinkholes in quick succession, likely openings into the same underground stream. Cross over the campground road and look for yellow blazes on the trees as you ascend the sandhills. Keep to the obvious path at the fork, where a small sinkhole is forming. Longleaf pines tower over wiregrass-covered hills where paw-paw blooms in spring. At 2.5 miles, you pass through a four-way junction of trails, transitioning into a hardwood hammock. Keep left at the next fork to walk down to Third Landing, a beauty spot overlooking marshes along Rock Springs Run.

Curve up to the T-intersection and turn left. Pass around the gate and cross the power line access road. Watch for the quick left turn and the yellow blazes as the trail becomes a pleasant corridor under deep shade, where bromeliads drape from the trees. After 3.1 miles, you emerge at the lower entrance to the swimming area and the back side of a **Kelly Loop Trail** sign. Turn left and walk past pavilion 3 to the boardwalk. It parallels Rock Springs Run downstream, with glimpses of the glassy waters. The boardwalk provides access to ramps into the water before crossing the stream. Past the next pavilion, keep right at the fork to walk through the bluff forest above the spring run. Stay left at the next fork or you'll end up in the middle of the main swimming area. Slash pines tower overhead, some with catface marks from turpentine tapping. Keep right at the next two forks to complete the loop. The trail drops back down through the lush forest to Rock Spring.

After you cross the bridge, wander down on the rocks on the left to peek into the cavern mouth in the hillside. The cavern is gated so no one can crawl into it, but you can look in and see the spring water flowing out. Retrace your steps back up the boardwalk to the main swimming and concession area to return to the parking area, completing the 4-mile hike.

Nearby Attractions

Since you've already paid to enter the park, be sure to cool off with a splash in this, Florida's prettiest natural water park. Snorkeling is permitted. You can bring your own tubes for the tubing run or rent them from a vendor at the corner of Rock Springs Road and Kelly Park Road. Paddlers can launch at Kings Landing for an expedition down Rock Springs Run to the Wekiva River: **kingslandingfl.com.**

Directions

From I-4 in Altamonte Springs, follow FL 436 (Semoran Boulevard) to Apopka, where it joins into US 441. Turn right onto Rock Springs Road (County Road 435). Drive 5.8 miles north to Kelly Park Road. You'll see a tube-rental stand on the corner. Turn right. Follow the road for less than 0.5 mile to the park entrance on the right. Pay your entrance fee at the ranger station and continue down the park entrance road to the main parking area. Park near the swimming area.

Lake Lotus Park

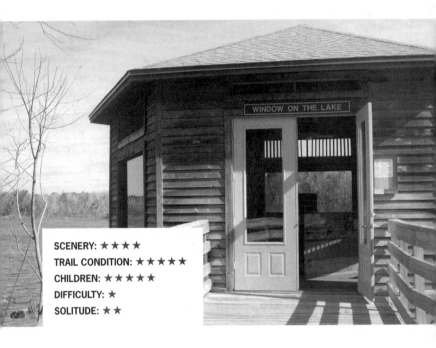

SCENERY: ★ ★ ★ ★
TRAIL CONDITION: ★ ★ ★ ★ ★
CHILDREN: ★ ★ ★ ★ ★
DIFFICULTY: ★
SOLITUDE: ★ ★

WINDOW ON THE LAKE OBSERVATION ROOM

GPS TRAILHEAD COORDINATES: N27° 22.413' W81° 58.679'

DISTANCE & CONFIGURATION: 1.2-mile loop

HIKING TIME: 40 minutes

HIGHLIGHTS: Wildlife-watching, big trees, marsh views

ACCESS: Free; open Thursday–Sunday, 8:30 a.m.–5:30 p.m.

MAPS: USGS *Forest City*

FACILITIES: Restrooms, playground, fishing pier, picnic pavilions

WHEELCHAIR ACCESS: Boardwalks are wheelchair accessible.

COMMENTS: The park gates are closed on weekends to avoid overcrowding in the small parking area. Use the external parking area, across Maitland Boulevard at Magnolia Homes Road, where a tram will take you into the park.

CONTACTS: Lake Lotus Park (407) 293-8885; **altamonte.org**

Overview

An unexpected treasure within densely packed suburban neighbor-hoods just north of Orlando, Lake Lotus Park is an urban woodland, protecting 150 acres of floodplain forest and pine flatwoods along its namesake lake and the upper reaches of the Little Wekiva River. Most of the trail system is made up of boardwalks with plenty of benches for young and old to rest, with a few natural-surface trails slipping deeper into the forest.

Route Details

Broad enough for two wheelchairs to pass, the boardwalk leaving the parking area is lined with tall cypresses. Turn right onto the side trail, which becomes a bark-chip path leading you along a narrow stream, the Little Wekiva River. Rising in the confusion of concrete and asphalt of Orlando to the west, this waterway broadens into Lake Lotus and flows out the other side of the lake, continuing beneath culverts and ditches through suburbia to eventually meet the Wekiva River in a wild floodplain. Past the benches, there is an interpretive display about the hydrology of the region. Turn left and walk to the overlook for a view of the winding stream.

At the park road, turn left to walk up toward the bridge. Make a right just before the bridge to follow the river upstream. At the T-intersection, turn right and enjoy the wonderland of the predomi-nant cinnamon and royal ferns, among other ferns, in the river flood-plain. Keep left at the fork. American beautyberry arcs over the trail, showing off its metallic-purple fruits. Large live oaks, laurel oaks, and water oaks make up the canopy of this shady forest, with dahoon holly, southern magnolia, and a scattering of cabbage palms. As the trail descends deeper into the floodplain, there is a tangle of large roots snaking around a red maple of enormous stature. The footpath may be squishy through this section, as muck and water rise through the dense layer of leaves. After 0.25 mile, the trail gains a little eleva-tion, just enough to change the soil underfoot. In a thicket of ferns,

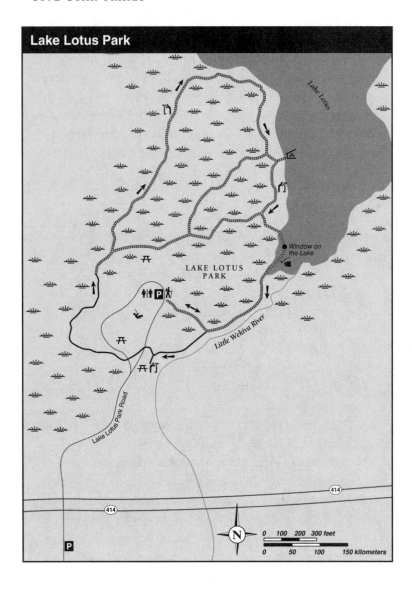

Lake Lotus Park

Lake Lotus

Window on the Lake

LAKE LOTUS PARK

Little Wekiva River

Lake Lotus Park Road

414

414

P

N

0   100   200   300 feet

0   50   100   150 kilometers

you pass citrus trees mixed into the floodplain forest, and an ephemeral waterway flows past on the left. At the T-intersection, there is a "You Are Here" map. Turn left. Netted chain fern grows closely along both edges of the footpath. More citrus trees, in full fruit in winter, are scattered through the floodplain. You reach the broad boardwalk, which is older and more uneven in character through this section. Ferns fill the understory beneath the tall cypresses and oaks.

At the junction in the boardwalk, turn left. Passing an interpretive sign about cypress trees, you emerge into the sunshine and walk through an open floodplain-forest habitat dense with Virginia willow. During the winter months, the red maples put on a fall foliage show through this section. The boardwalk ducks into the shade of a canopy of laurel oaks as it comes to a large observation deck with benches. Zigzagging above the marshy ground, it continues toward Lake Lotus. Duck beneath a low live oak limb as the boardwalk turns right and heads down a straightaway. By 0.7 mile, you see a broad marsh where wading birds stay near shore and coots gather in bobbing flocks on the water. Carpeted with American lotus, the marsh is especially pretty in summer when these floating lilies are in bloom.

The boardwalk continues around the bend to meet the open waters of Lake Lotus, edged by apartments on the far shore. Swinging to the right, it remains in the shade as you reach the next T-intersection. Turn left to walk down to the Window on the Lake. This observation room has interpretive information and is a virtual blind from which you can watch the birds, alligators, and turtles without disturbing them. As you leave the Window on the Lake, turn left, passing another observation deck.

At the next trail junction, turn left. This boardwalk arcs out over the open water and provides the best wildlife viewing in the park. Look closely—alligators often blend right into the vegetation in the shallows. A purple gallinule and its chicks hop between lily pads. The boardwalk broadens to create a wheelchair-accessible fishing area. Along the shoreline, swamp sunflowers paint a scene against the backdrop of colors in the floodplain forest each fall.

Leaving the lake as you continue along the boardwalk, you follow the Little Wekiva River upstream for a short segment. As you pass a quartet of cypresses, you complete the loop. Continue straight ahead to exit the boardwalk to the parking area, finishing your hike near the playground and restrooms after 1.2 miles.

Nearby Attractions

The stylized Mayan temple motif of the 1930s-era Maitland Art Center invites you to explore its courtyards and working artist studios. It anchors a complex of historic buildings: **artandhistory.org.** See raptors in rehab at the Audubon Center for Birds of Prey: **fl.audubon.org /audubon-center-birds-prey.**

Directions

From I-4, follow FL 414 (Maitland Boulevard) west for 2.7 miles, passing Maitland Center and the FL 434 interchange. The next traffic light leads you into Lake Lotus Park (on the right) or to Magnolia Homes Road (on the left) for the weekend overflow parking area. Follow the park road all the way to where it starts to loop around the playground, and park near the picnic pavilions and restroom.

Seminole State Forest: Lower Wekiva Loop

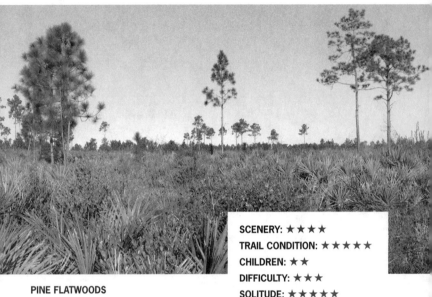

SCENERY: ★ ★ ★ ★
TRAIL CONDITION: ★ ★ ★ ★ ★
CHILDREN: ★ ★
DIFFICULTY: ★ ★ ★
SOLITUDE: ★ ★ ★ ★

PINE FLATWOODS

GPS TRAILHEAD COORDINATES: N28° 49.152' W81° 25.683'

DISTANCE & CONFIGURATION: 8.8-mile loop

HIKING TIME: 4½ hours

HIGHLIGHTS: Vast panoramic views, ancient trees, wildflowers

ACCESS: $2 per person; open 24/7

MAPS: USGS *Sanford SW*

FACILITIES: Privies and picnic pavilion at Bear Pond Trailhead, trail shelter, primitive campsite with picnic table and fire ring

WHEELCHAIR ACCESS: None

COMMENTS: Excellent habitat for Florida black bear and Florida scrub-jays

CONTACTS: Florida Forest Service, Leesburg Forestry Station (352) 360-6675 or (352) 360-6677; **floridaforestservice.com/state_forests**

Seminole State Forest: Lower Wekiva Loop

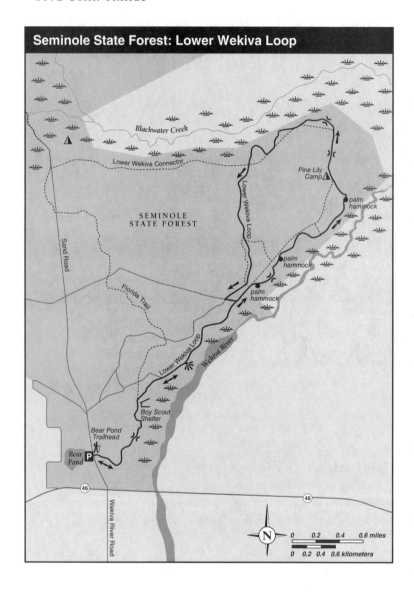

Overview

A lesser-known but beautiful loop trail within Seminole State Forest, the Lower Wekiva Loop traces the edge of both the Wekiva River and Blackwater Creek to where the waters merge. This 8.8-mile loop never gets within sight of either waterway but lingers in spectacular palm hammocks in the lowlands, showcasing ancient trees and colorful wildflowers such as the pine lily. Traversing open scrub, sandhills, and pine savanna habitats, it also offers a counterpoint of expansive views against the lush intimacy of the hammocks. With a footpath built and maintained by the Florida Trail Association, it's a fine example of trail craftsmanship.

Route Details

From the Bear Pond Trailhead, follow the **Florida Trail** north. After 0.5 mile, the trail crosses a bridge in the deep shade of a hardwood hammock before it rises up and broadens to a grassy corridor. Climbing up through scrubby flatwoods, you encounter the Boy Scout shelter on the edge of an expansive scrub forest. Just past the shelter, turn right to come to the well-marked junction of the **Florida Trail** with the **Lower Wekiva Loop,** at 0.9 mile. Turn right.

Marked with white blazes, the **Lower Wekiva Loop** starts out in the scrub forest. This low scrub is ideal for Florida scrub-jays, bright-blue birds which are only found in Florida and are frequently seen along this section of trail amid the soft, fluffy young sand pines, myrtle oak, and Chapman oak. After 1.4 miles, you pass a firebreak to the left at the edge of the scrub and enter a tunnel under the sand live oaks. You can see tall cypresses and palms outlining the meandering flow of the Wekiva River in the distance, but you can't get there from here, even at the gentle fork in the trail just past a firebreak. Keep left. A pine savanna stretches off to the right, with spindly, bristly pond pines reaching for the broad skies above. Diving into a scrub corridor and emerging again into the sunlight, the trail slips along the vast savanna.

At 2.2 miles, the next trail on the left is where you'll return later to complete this loop. It connects to the equestrian trail system through this part of the forest. Continue straight. Descending under tall slash pines, the footpath hits a short rolling section where sweetgum shades the trail. Low spots can become damp at times. Clambering atop an old logging tramway, look off to the left at the expanse of pine savanna. As you leave the tramway, it's a steady descent to reach the first dense hammock along the river basin. The cabbage palms that rise overhead are ancient, with clumped rootballs smothered in sphagnum moss reaching up to waist height. Glossy, dark-leaved needle palms are scattered throughout the understory. A bridge crosses an ephemeral stream that flows out to the Wekiva River. After winding beneath curving palms, the trail rises back up to the pine savanna and then enters the scrub, with low trees perfect for scrub-jays and lots of gallberry. The trail works its way through pine flatwoods and scrub, passing tall, spindly slash pines, and drops into a palm hammock to jog past a wet prairie, a good place to see pine lilies in summer. Cabbage palms and live oaks tower overhead, knitting a high canopy as the trail continues its descent, this time toward the floodplain of Blackwater Creek, which flows into the Wekiva River.

Reaching an old forest road at 3.8 miles, the trail turns right. Follow the white blazes. A blue-blazed trail to the left leads to Pine Lily Camp, a pretty, primitive campsite deep within a palm hammock. Continue along the trail to cross a boardwalk paralleling the road. Blue flag iris sprouts from the swales and puts on a beautiful show in the springtime. Keep alert as you walk down this straightaway, since the trail leaves it at a sharp left at 4.4 miles and an unmarked path keeps going straight ahead. Loblolly pine surrounds the trail, and there are many bromeliads overhead in the limbs of the old live oaks, enjoying the humidity of the high canopy. After crossing another bridge over an ephemeral stream, the corridor becomes broad and comfortable enough to walk three abreast, although it is not a forest road. In the winter, you can look off to the right and see the floodplain forest of Blackwater Creek through the lower canopy.

At 4.8 miles, you transition from palm hammock into pine flat-woods. A small floodplain swamp sits off to the left. Saw palmetto rises to shoulder height along this broad trail. Passing through the shade of an oak hammock, the trail quickly curves back out into the pines again. You ascend to a major trail junction at 5.4 miles. This junction marks the official end of the hiking-only Lower Wekiva Loop. However, you can use the multiuse equestrian trails to make a full loop out of this hike. To the right, the trail goes off to meet the **Florida Trail** near Blackwater Creek (Hike 30, page 195).

Turn left to start following the equestrian trail to complete the loop. This is a broad forest road with easy walking and scattered shade. After a shaded corridor, the path rises into pond pine flat-woods with very little shade. Colorful grasses fill the gaps between saw palmetto in the understory, including lovegrass in a pink hue. At 6 miles, there is a junction with a yellow-tipped post and green

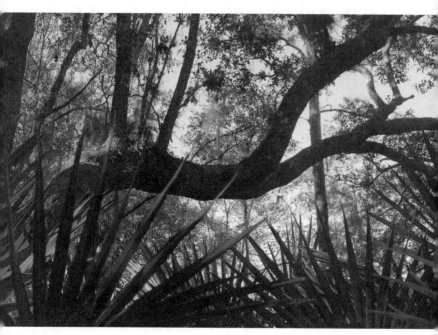

LIVE OAK ABOVE THE SAW PALMETTO

markers pointing off to the right. Continue walking straight ahead. At the next fork, keep to the right, following the arrow into an open pine savanna with wiregrass and the skinny slash pines. It's a long walk across this expanse, with beautiful views the whole way.

Reaching a four-way trail junction at 6.6 miles in a sandy spot, turn left. The pines on your left are oddly curved. Follow this forest road. As it curves to the left, look for a marker with a NO HORSES symbol on the right. It leads to a footpath, partially blocked by deadfall, which connects you right back to the Lower Wekiva Loop. Turn right. Walking back down the corridor of fluffy sand pines, be alert for Florida scrub-jays. You reach the junction with the **Florida Trail** and its trail register at 7.9 miles. Turn left. Passing the Boy Scout shelter, continue along the orange-blazed **Florida Trail** as it follows the broad corridor through the pine flatwoods and narrows down before it crosses the bridge. Continue back to the **Bear Pond Trailhead,** completing your hike after 8.8 miles.

Nearby Attractions

The Florida Trail through Seminole State Forest (Hike 30, page 195) shares the trail for the southernmost mile. Seminole State Forest touches several other public lands with hiking trails that are not covered by this book, including Lower Wekiva River Preserve State Park and Rock Springs Run Reserve State Park, both accessible from FL 46: **floridastateparks.org.** Just east of the trailhead entrance, Wekiva Falls RV Resort offers water slides, canoeing, and kayaking: **wekiva fallsresort.com.**

Directions

From I-4, Exit 101C at Sanford, take FL 46 west for 5.2 miles. After you cross the Wekiva River, look for the entrance to Seminole State Forest on the right. Continue 1 mile along the forest road—stopping at the self-service kiosk to pay the day-use fee—to park on the left.

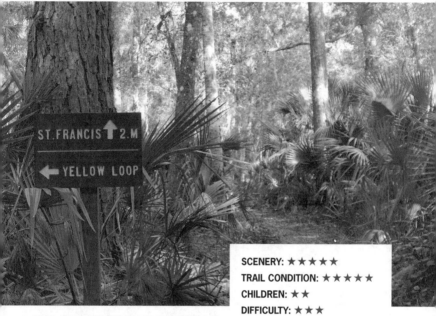

ST.FRANCIS ↑ 2.M

← YELLOW LOOP

SCENERY: ★ ★ ★ ★ ★
TRAIL CONDITION: ★ ★ ★ ★ ★
CHILDREN: ★ ★
DIFFICULTY: ★ ★ ★
SOLITUDE: ★ ★ ★ ★ ★

TRAIL JUNCTION ON THE ST. FRANCIS LOOP

GPS TRAILHEAD COORDINATES: N29° 0.769' W81° 23.545'

DISTANCE & CONFIGURATION: 7.9-mile balloon

HIKING TIME: 4 hours

HIGHLIGHTS: Ancient trees, river views, unusual fungi

ACCESS: Free; open 24/7

MAPS: USGS *Lake Woodruff*

FACILITIES: None

WHEELCHAIR ACCESS: None

COMMENTS: Trail will flood if the St. Johns River is high. Primitive camping permitted, except during hunting season. Leashed pets welcome.

CONTACTS: Ocala National Forest, Seminole Ranger District (352) 669-3153; **fs.usda.gov/ocala**

St. Francis Trail

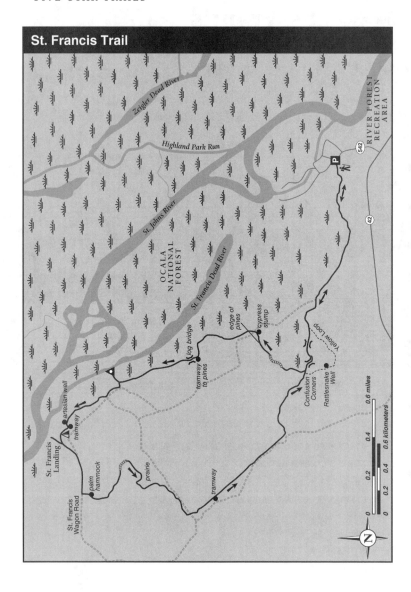

Overview

One of the region's most scenic and easy-to-follow day hikes, the St. Francis Trail traverses the southeastern corner of the Ocala National Forest to lead you through what was once farms, fields, and a bustling commercial center in the late 1800s. It's hard to believe, as you walk through the deep shade under live oaks and cabbage palms, that a town once crowded the wharf where the St. Johns River turns away from the St. Francis Dead River. Bounded by the Alexander Springs Wilderness and the floodplain forests of the mighty St. Johns River, this is a wild and wonderful wander.

Route Details

Starting at the trailhead kiosk, where you'll learn about St. Francis's agricultural past, follow the orange blazes into an upland hammock of oaks. The footpath is well defined and easy to follow as you amble through this shady second-growth forest. Crossing a short bridge, the trail turns left to tunnel into the woods. Despite the size of the trees, there are clues that this was once a farmer's field. You can see the wavy shapes of furrows on either side, the forest growing atop the undulations. There are mats in some of the dips, placed there long ago by trail maintainers to help stop erosion.

After the next small bridge, a long boardwalk begins, covered in hardware cloth to help keep you from slipping. Thanks to the constant humidity, ferns and fungi are prolific. Colonies of collybia mushrooms spill out of rotten stumps; violet cort and coral fungus emerge from leaf litter. Your surroundings feel primordial, and you'll hike this part twice. After crossing a bridge over a tannic waterway, you come to the first junction with the **Yellow Loop** at a sign at 1.2 miles. Continue straight ahead. After the next bridge, you reach Confusion Corners, where there are three trail junctions in quick succession. The first one, on the right, has a sign that says ST. FRANCIS, 2 MILES. Turn right at the sign.

Walking counterclockwise around the loop gets you closer to the river more quickly, which is evident as you walk through lush cabbage palm hammocks where sunlight filters through the fronds to create an illuminating glow. Boardwalks carry you over damp areas. Rising uphill, the trail skims the edge of a pine forest. It continues to wobble back and forth, in the pines one moment and back into the palms the next. Crossing a bridge over a murky stream, you enter an oak hammock with a pine plantation atop the hill. This was likely one of the last areas farmed in St. Francis before the U.S. Forest Service took over the land in the 1940s and planted pines.

After 2.4 miles, the trail scrambles up a levee to reach a log bridge over a creek. Use the guylines to help keep your footing as you cross this bridge. Bowls of saw palmetto sweep off to the right as the trail dips low to go around a large fallen tree. You see cypresses, an indication that the river is near. Water often collects in the footpath through this section. Palm fronds dip right across the trail, making the hike feel like a jungle exploration. When the path straightens out, you're following an old tramway through the swamp.

At a T-intersection with a sandy path with tannic water flowing across it, the blazes lead left, but you'll want to turn right for a short detour. This spur tramway burrows through a low canopy of palms to emerge at the St. Francis Dead River. Fossilized snail shells spill off the bank. At 3 miles, it's a pretty overlook. Return the way you came and turn right at the fork. The trail immediately turns right again to continue through the floodplain. You pass a continually flowing artesian well that pours out of a pipe into an overflowing barrel. It's off the trail, but you can find it easily by the sound and the smell of sulfur in the air.

You reach the St. Francis Road at a T-intersection after 3.7 miles. This was Main Street for the town, with a post office, general store, and residences along both sides of a wagon road leading to Paisley. Take a short ramble down to the right to the end of the road, where you can see the pilings from the old wharf along the St. Johns River. Turn around and follow the orange blazes along the road. Since it sits lower than the surrounding landscape, expect large puddles to skirt or wade through. Within 0.3 mile, the trail veers off the road and left into the forest, working its way through cabbage palms and large live oaks.

As the elevation increases, slash pines and pond pines create a sparse canopy, while saw palmetto fills the understory. Despite the dense thickets of saw palmetto, the footpath is smooth and strewn with pine duff. Dipping in and out of shady spots, there are places where you can see for some distance across the pine flatwoods. Crossing several jeep trails, the trail works its way along a bayhead swamp where water may trickle into the footpath. You reach another logging tramway at 5.8 miles. The trail follows the tramway through bayhead swamps, veering off in several places to avoid areas that collect deep standing water. Crossing several more jeep trails, the trail returns to Confusion Corners, where you enter a clearing under the oaks with a sign for the **Yellow Loop** off to your right. Turn right to amble back along this short side trail.

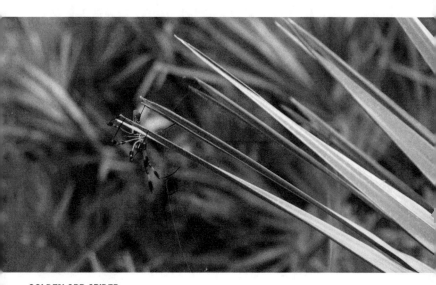

GOLDEN ORB SPIDER

A long boardwalk leads over a grassy area thick with ferns. After crossing two short bridges, you drop down a slope to cross a steeply eroded creek. The trail turns left to follow this small creek under a stand of southern magnolias. You cross several more bridges as the trail meanders through oak hammocks to its main point of interest, Rattlesnake Well. This sulfuric spring is a swirling hole of turquoise blue with yellow streamers, mesmerizing and smelly. Continue a short distance and you reach the main trail again at a T-intersection. You've walked 6.7 miles. Turn right to head back down the entrance trail you came in on to wrap up a 7.9-mile hike when you reach the trailhead.

Nearby Attractions

Historic downtown DeLand (**mainstreetdeland.org**) has an eclectic collection of galleries and museums, among them the Gillespie Museum of Minerals at Stetson University (**stetson.edu/other /gillespie**), which contains one of the oldest and largest mineral collections in the Southeast.

Directions

From DeLand, drive north on FL 15 or US 17 to intersect with FL 44. Head west on FL 44 (New York Avenue) for 4.2 miles from FL 15, crossing the Whitehair Bridge over the St. Johns River. Turn right onto FL 42 at the light after the bridge. Watch for the sign on the right; it comes up fast. Turn right at River Forest and drive past the group camp to the trailhead at the end of this short, unpaved road.

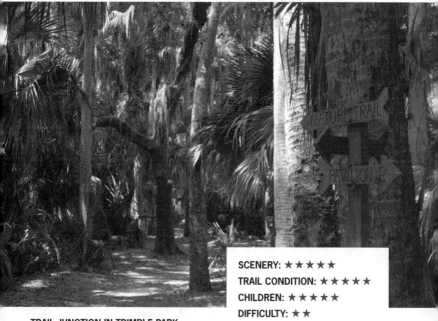

SCENERY: ★ ★ ★ ★ ★
TRAIL CONDITION: ★ ★ ★ ★ ★
CHILDREN: ★ ★ ★ ★ ★
DIFFICULTY: ★ ★
SOLITUDE: ★ ★ ★

TRAIL JUNCTION IN TRIMBLE PARK

GPS TRAILHEAD COORDINATES: N28° 45.940' W81° 39.114'

DISTANCE & CONFIGURATION: 1.3-mile loop

HIKING TIME: 45 minutes

HIGHLIGHTS: Ancient oaks and cypresses, constant breezes, excellent birding

ACCESS: Free; open daily, 8 a.m.–8 p.m. in summer; open daily, 8 a.m.–6 p.m. in winter

MAPS: USGS *Eustis*

FACILITIES: Restrooms, playgrounds, boat ramp, picnic pavilions, fishing pier, campground

WHEELCHAIR ACCESS: Limited to boardwalk sections

COMMENTS: A campground that accommodates both group tent camping and trailers is set around a small cove along the lake. There are many shorter options to hiking this loop.

CONTACTS: Trimble Park (352) 383-1993; **apps.ocfl.net/dept/cesrvcs/parks/ParkDetails .asp?ParkID=40**

Trimble Park

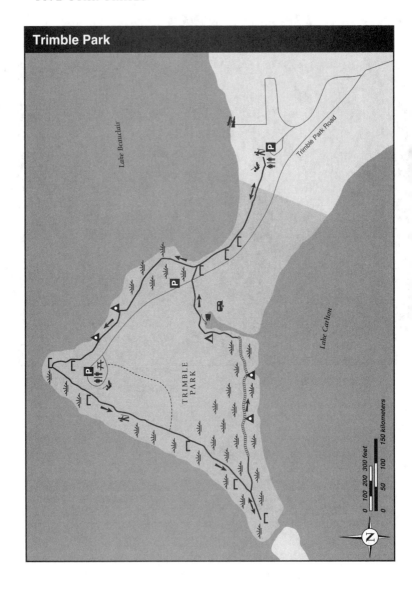

Lake Beauclair

Trimble Park Road

Lake Carlton

TRIMBLE
PARK

0 100 200 300 feet
0   50   100   150 kilometers

Overview

At the end of a 71-acre peninsula between Lake Beauclair and Lake Carlton in the Harris chain of lakes, Trimble Park is an under-the-radar beauty spot of which Orange County should be quite proud. Ancient oaks shade the picnic grove and playground at the end of the road where most visitors gravitate. This 1.3-mile loop follows the shoreline on pathways, a nature trail, and boardwalks under tall cypresses and live oaks.

Route Details

From the boat ramp parking area, walk up to the playground. Keep left to walk along a shaded gravel path. Above you are mature wild citrus trees, dripping with fruit or fragrant blooms. Paralleling the park road, the trail comes to an intersection. Keep right at the fork. Coots squawk as they dart in and out of stands of pickerelweed in Lake Beauclair. Just after passing a side trail, you reach a bench overlooking the water. Walking a short distance, you encounter two more benches waiting for you to sit and watch the birds. A sign pointing toward the campground indicates you've reached the beginning of the loop. Continue straight ahead, passing a picnic table.

Notice how immense the cypresses are along the shoreline of Lake Beauclair. This side of the park seems more abundant in bird life, especially in the morning. Slipping past benches, picnic tables, and even a barbecue grill, don't forget to be alert for alligators. The shoreline is such a gentle slope that an alligator could easily be sunning in the footpath, which stays close to the water. Look for turtles on the logs near shore.

Philodendrons with massive leaves climb the ancient oaks, creating a junglelike feel. The trail ascends a berm. Cabbage palms tower overhead, and moss-draped oaks arc out over the water. Headed downhill through a patch of sword fern, you can see the park road off to your left. Keep to the right to follow the trail. You come to a boat ramp with an observation deck adjoining it, where a cormorant might be drying its wings in the sun. This observation point provides a sweeping view along the peninsula.

The path isn't as obvious beyond this point, so follow the shoreline. A fishing pier protrudes into the lake, providing perches for great blue herons and more cormorants. Follow the sweep of the lakeshore to the point of the peninsula, where there are benches and swings for contemplating the scenery and a marshy area with many wading birds. Continue around the shoreline past the marsh, passing the main picnic shelters, playground, and restrooms under the ancient live oaks.

After 0.5 mile, you reach a junction with a boardwalk from a picnic shelter and the **Nature Trail** sign. Continue straight ahead down a corridor framed by cabbage palms and wild citrus. The breeze off the lakes makes this a cool walk, despite the thickness of the understory. There are many roots underfoot, so be cautious of your footing. On the left is a tangle of floodplain forest with sweetgum and red maple trees. At the next trail junction, continue straight. Sunlight dapples through the palm fronds across a bench. Peek through the understory for glimpses of the cattail marsh along the lake.

At the next junction, signs say THE POINT to the right and BOARDWALK to the left. Turn right. Wild coffee grows thickly in the understory. Oaks reach out over the lake's edge. At the T-intersection, turn right again to continue to The Point, the meeting place of Lake Beauclair and Lake Carlton through a narrow canal that was dug through an isthmus a long time ago. A bench provides a view. Retrace your steps to the intersection. At the trail junction, keep to the right, following the sign that says BOARDWALK.

Elevation drops as the trail winds through palm hammock. At the next trail junction, continue straight ahead to start the boardwalk. At 0.9 mile a glider bench looks out over a profusion of ferns and reeds. Large cypresses shade this section of the boardwalk as you walk along it, reaching an open platform, a beauty spot overlooking Lake Carlton. At the next junction, cattails crowd close to the trail.

Continue straight ahead. Sunlight pours into gaps in the canopy. To your right is another observation deck. Passing the next junction, continue straight ahead.

A stand of cypresses shades the end of the boardwalk, which faces a small cove. Turn left to walk along this cove, passing the kayak launch and the group campground. Walk through the gap in the fence. Circling the cove, you encounter some fishing platforms. Beyond them is the park's deeply shaded campground. At the CAMP-ERS ONLY sign, keep left to walk through the next gap in the fence into the parking area. Cross the parking area and the park road. Head down the slope to Lake Beauclair and turn right. Following the berm, you return to the original loop junction. Step off to the left, by the bench, and take the footpath along the lake. It provides one last opportunity for birding as you walk back to the parking area, completing your hike after 1.3 miles.

Nearby Attractions

Mount Dora, 4 miles north, is Florida's antiquing capital. The unusually hilly historic village sweeps down to the shores of Lake Dora: **mountdora.com.**

Directions

From the intersection of Lake Ola Drive and US 441 near Zellwood, turn left on Lake Ola Drive and continue not quite a mile to Earlwood Avenue. Turn left. After 0.7 mile, make a right onto Trimble Park Road. Entering the park, immediately make a right at the park office into the first parking area, which has a boat ramp and restrooms; park near the playground. There are also several parking areas along the trail route, deeper inside the park.

Wekiwa Springs Hiking Trail

SCENERY: ★ ★ ★ ★ ★
TRAIL CONDITION: ★ ★ ★ ★
CHILDREN: ★ ★ ★
DIFFICULTY: ★ ★ ★ ★
SOLITUDE: ★ ★ ★ ★

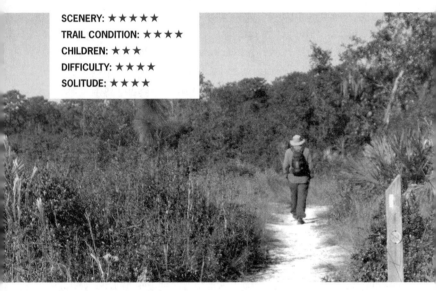

HIKING INTO THE SCRUBBY UPLANDS OF WEKIWA SPRINGS STATE PARK

GPS TRAILHEAD COORDINATES: N28° 43.425' W81° 28.395'

DISTANCE & CONFIGURATION: 10.8-mile loop

HIKING TIME: 6.5 hours

HIGHLIGHTS: Expansive rolling landscapes, spring and fall wildflowers, cypress swamps, views of Rock Springs Run

ACCESS: State park entrance fee of $2 per pedestrian or bicyclist, $4 per individual driver, $6 for 2–8 people in a vehicle; open daily, 8 a.m.–sunset

MAPS: USGS *Forest City* and *Apopka;* trail map at ranger station

FACILITIES: Restrooms, picnic areas, campground, nature center, youth camp, canoe and kayak rentals, guided horseback rides, swimming area with concession

WHEELCHAIR ACCESS: None

COMMENTS: Leave plenty of time to complete the loop. Shorter options are available; refer to the park map. Parts of the trail are shared with off-road cyclists and equestrians. Insect repellent is a must. Leashed dogs permitted. The park is

busy on summer weekends and will close the gates when maximum capacity
for parking is reached.

CONTACTS: Wekiwa Springs State Park (407) 884-2008; **floridastateparks.org
/wekiwasprings**

Overview

More than a million people live within 20 miles of Wekiwa Springs
State Park, where Orlando's suburban sprawl encroaches from several directions. It's one of Florida's busiest and most popular state
parks, with Wekiwa Springs the primary destination for most visitors. With more than 42,000 acres protected along the federally
designated Wild and Scenic River basin among several adjoining
state parks, this is a truly wild place. You'll sample the wilderness
along the Wekiwa Springs Hiking Trail. This extensive trail system
transports you to a different world, far from the hubbub of campers
and swimmers, immersing you in vast landscapes where deer and
Florida black bear roam.

Route Details

From the Sand Lake Trailhead, walk up the sidewalk through the low
scrub forest, passing the restrooms to reach a trail junction at marker
23. Numbered markers appear all along this hike, making it easier for
park personnel to find lost hikers. Continue straight ahead to start
walking clockwise around the loop, following the white blazes. The
trail descends into an oak scrub. Keep left at the fork, as the trail
drops down into a floodplain forest. Reaching a junction with an
orange-blazed trail at a bench, follow the white blazes as they guide
you away from the park road and into a tunnel under the oaks. As
the trail drops down to the edge of the floodplain forest, ferns fill the
understory, and the air becomes markedly cooler. Traversing a bridge,
the trail—now blazed orange, yellow, and white—ascends through
several habitats before reaching sandhills with an open understory.
You may spot deer dashing across the footpath.

Wekiwa Springs Hiking Trail

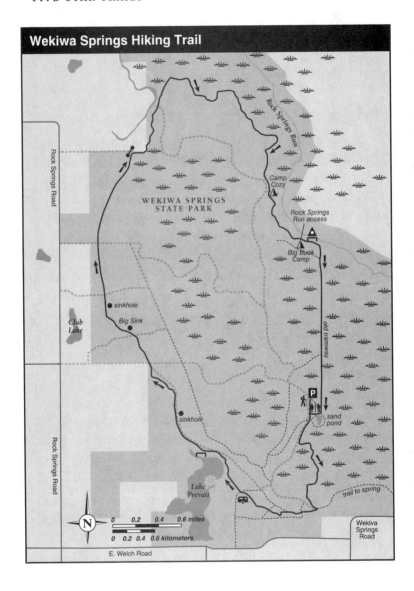

Rock Springs Road

WEKIWA SPRINGS
STATE PARK

Rock Springs Run

Camp
Cozy

Rock Springs
Run access

Big Buck
Camp

old tramway

sinkhole

Big Sink

Club
Lake

sinkhole

P

sand
pond

Lake
Prevatt

trail to spring

Rock Springs Road

N

| 0 | 0.2 | 0.4 | 0.6 miles |

| 0 | 0.2 | 0.4 | 0.6 kilometers |

Wekiva
Springs
Road

E. Welch Road

Following a small ridge above the floodplain of the Wekiva River, the trail reaches a major junction at 1.1 miles. Straight ahead, the footpath leads to the springs. Turn right, and ignore the mileages posted on the sign: they're missing decimal points. Cross the park road to follow orange and white blazes beneath the longleaf pines. Past the campground, you cross the campground road and the road to Camp Wekiva in quick succession. The trail drops steeply through the forest to circle around Lake Prevatt, which is revealed only by glimpses through the trees. You can hear moorhens along the shoreline but saw palmetto blocks the view. A bench sits above the lake at 2.5 miles but has no view of the water.

The next major trail junction is at marker 10. The orange blazes turn right, blue blazes pass by, and red blazes join the white blazes ahead of you, indicating this section of trail is shared with mountain bikes. A big sinkhole sits off to the right, with saw palmetto and mature trees growing from the bottom. At 3.5 miles, the trail crosses a power line road with a bench just beyond the crossing. As you climb the low ridges of the sandhills, coastal plain palafox engulfs the trail in a sea of fragrant white blossoms each fall. Soon after marker 12, there is a side trail to a very large and deep sinkhole. As the habitat transitions into hardwood forest, the trail slopes downhill, skirting a small sinkhole before rising into another expansive stretch of sandhills. By 4.6 miles, you can see a nursery in the distance as the trail pulls within sight of the park boundary fence.

After traversing another panoramic landscape, the trail comes to a bench in the shade. The understory closes in, and you must push through saw palmetto fronds to reach the next expanse of sandhills. Passing marker 17 at a green-blazed horse trail, the trail winds past an open pine savanna and rounds a bayhead swamp, reaching a back gate to the park at 5.5 miles. Heading downhill fast, with red, green, and white blazes on the trees, you enter a cypress swamp. Thick mud tries to wrench off your shoes. At the next bench, make sure you spray yourself liberally with insect repellent. Marker 19 is where the mountain bike and equestrian trails depart, while the white blazes guide you deeper into the swampy floodplain of Rock Springs Run. Although you can't see it, you're very close to the Kelly Loop Trail at Kelly Park (Hike 32, page 206).

Crossing a bridge that might not span far enough to cross the swiftly flowing stream, the trail drops into deep mud. Ancient oaks tower overhead, creating a high canopy, and palm fronds slap you in the face. As you can tell from the condition of the footpath, the adjacent waterway frequently swamps the trail. After the next bridge, you walk down a corridor darkened by the glistening fronds of needle palms. Around marker 19B, look up and notice the sheer size of the trees around you, true ancients of the forest. Tulip poplar, near the southern extent of its range, is among them. Wild coffee grows in the mucky, wet understory. The trail becomes a little indistinct within this riot of greenery, a tight and tricky corridor under the palms. Keep looking for the next white blaze. For the next 0.5 mile, the trail weaves back and forth between wet and dry habitats, reaching an ancient and stately palm hammock around 7 miles, with a second one a little farther down the trail.

The cool shade dissipates as the trail ascends into scrubby pond pine flatwoods, the footpath now level, solid, and without roots in the way. Passing a bench, you come to Camp Cozy, a primitive campsite at 7.8 miles with a fire ring surrounded by benches and a spigot with nonpotable water. Continuing through the camp, the trail crosses a stream as it descends into sloppy, muddy goop along the floodplain of Rock Springs Run. Mosquitoes buzz in swarms. At 8.4 miles, the trail reaches a forest road. To the left, you can walk down to Rock Springs Run. The trail turns right and ascends to Big Buck Camp, another primitive campsite with picnic tables, a fire ring, and nonpotable water. As the trail leaves the camp, it winds through a dense palm hammock with cypress knees underfoot. Finally, you reach a bench with a view of Rock Springs Run. Sit and savor this hard-won view. The trail ever-so-briefly continues within sight of the waterway before it enters another maze of cypress knees and turns away from the run, heading uphill.

Reaching marker 21 at a junction with a forest road and a double blaze, don't make the turn. Continue straight ahead into deep shade, following the trail up an old logging tramway into the floodplain forest. Sluggish waters spread across the swamp on both sides. You can see a fair distance ahead. A tricky, makeshift balance beam of a bridge gets you over a cut through the tramway where the tannic water flows through. A more substantial bridge is just beyond it.

Soon after the trail bursts out into sunlight, you reach the intersection with the **East-West Cross Trail** at 9.5 miles. Continue straight ahead, following the white blazes across Mill Creek on an old bridge. Bamboo crowds the footpath. The corridor widens significantly from tramway to forest road width, quickly rising up to a T-intersection at 10 miles. Look to the right, and you can see the restrooms at Sand Lake in the distance. Turn right. Keep to the left at the fork. Passing Sand Lake, you see benches on the far side, overlooking the scenic view. Reaching marker 23, you've completed the loop. Turn right and walk past the restrooms, down the sidewalk, and back to the parking area, finishing the 10.8-mile hike.

Nearby Attractions

Wekiwa Springs State Park is a destination in itself. Since the above route does not take you to the spring basin, make a point of visiting it after your hike. It's a great place to cool off after a day on the trail. Located next to the nature center at the springs, Wekiwa Springs State Park Nature Adventures can set you up with a canoe or kayak to explore the river or with a guided trail ride on the equestrian trails: **canoewekiva.com.**

Directions

From I-4, Exit 94, follow FL 434 west for 1 mile to Wekiwa Springs Road. Turn right. Drive 4.1 miles to the park entrance on the right. Once you pay your admission fee, take the left fork of the park road and follow it to where it ends at Sand Lake Trailhead.

Appendix A: Outdoor Retailers

While many outlets—from drugstores to supercenters—carry items that would be useful on the trail, the following retailers carry hiking gear. The oldest outfitter in the region, Travel Country Outdoors, draws hikers from around the state because of its very specific hiking and backpacking focus.

BASS PRO SHOPS
5156 International Drive
Orlando, FL 32819
(800) 227-7776
basspro.com

MOSQUITO CREEK OUTDOORS
170 South Washington Avenue
Apopka, FL 32703
(407) 464-2000
mosquitocreekoutdoors.com

GANDER MOUNTAIN
3750 Flagg Lane
Lake Mary, FL 32746
(407) 804-0514
gandermountain.com

TRAVEL COUNTRY OUTDOORS
1101 East Altamonte Drive
Altamonte Springs, FL 32701
(407) 831-0777
travelcountry.com

Appendix B: Map Resources

General

Visitor centers and ranger stations generally provide free maps of the trails in their areas.

Five-Star Trails: Orlando guidebook

Download GPS tracks of the trails in this book at **floridahikes.com/5starorlando.**

Appendix C: Hiking Clubs

The clubs listed below have long, stable histories and welcome visitors to their meetings. All clubs welcome nonmembers to their meetings and to some of their activities.

CENTRAL FLORIDA SIERRA CLUB

P.O. Box 941692
Maitland, FL 32794-1692
centralfloridasierra.org
Annual dues: $39 (for nationwide membership)
Meetings are held on the third Wednesday of each month at 6:30 p.m. at Harry P. Leu Gardens, Orlando.

FLORIDA TRAIL ASSOCIATION/CENTRAL FLORIDA CHAPTER

510 Barclay Avenue
Altamonte Springs, FL 32701
meetup.com/Florida-Trail-Association-Central-Florida-Chapter
Annual dues: $30–35 (for statewide membership)
Contact: Jean Williamson, Membership Coordinator: jwilliamson3@cfl.rr.com
Meetings are held on the second Thursday of each month at 6:30 p.m. at Harry P. Leu Gardens, Orlando.

FLORIDA TRAIL ASSOCIATION/INDIAN RIVER CHAPTER

P.O. Box 832
Melbourne, FL 32902
meetup.com/SpaceCoastHiking
Annual dues: $30–35 (for statewide membership)
Contact: Richard Louden: lindaglouden@cfl.rr.com
Meetings are held on the first Monday of each month at 6:30 p.m. at the Melbourne Public Library.

ORLANDO-AREA HIKERS NETWORK

hiking.meetup.com/cities/us/fl/orlando

Index

About the Author

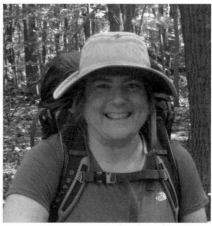

photographed by John Keatley

A hiker since she was old enough to toddle through the Appalachians with her parents, Sandra Friend is known as Florida's hiking expert. She has tallied more than 3,000 miles on foot throughout the state. Hiking, paddling, backpacking, and rafting are all a part of her outdoor résumé, which she expects to expand upon greatly in the years ahead with the outdoorsy man in her life.

Known best for her nature writing, Sandra is also a travel writer. A member of the Society of American Travel Writers and the Florida Outdoor Writers Association, she has authored 27 books since 1999, more than half of them about her home state of Florida. Her off-trail excursions involve immersing herself in historic places, driving back roads to find rural treasures, and visiting public gardens. Always curious about the natural world, she'll go miles out of her way to see a waterfall, a sinkhole, or an outcrop of minerals.

An avid photographer, Sandra enjoys sharing her outdoor experiences around the world, from the mountaintops of Nepal to the Patagonian steppes. Follow Sandra's adventures at **floridahikes.com** and **buckettripper.com.**

DEAR CUSTOMERS AND FRIENDS,

SUPPORTING YOUR INTEREST IN OUTDOOR ADVENTURE, travel, and an active lifestyle is central to our operations, from the authors we choose to the locations we detail to the way we design our books. Menasha Ridge Press was incorporated in 1982 by a group of veteran outdoorsmen and professional outfitters. For many years now, we've specialized in creating books that benefit the outdoors enthusiast.

Almost immediately, Menasha Ridge Press earned a reputation for revolutionizing outdoors- and travel-guidebook publishing. For such activities as canoeing, kayaking, hiking, backpacking, and mountain biking, we established new standards of quality that transformed the whole genre, resulting in outdoor-recreation guides of great sophistication and solid content. Menasha Ridge continues to be outdoor publishing's greatest innovator.

The folks at Menasha Ridge Press are as at home on a white-water river or mountain trail as they are editing a manuscript. The books we build for you are the best they can be, because we're responding to your needs. Plus, we use and depend on them ourselves.

We look forward to seeing you on the river or the trail. If you'd like to contact us directly, join in at www.trekalong.com or visit us at www.menasharidge.com. We thank you for your interest in our books and the natural world around us all.

SAFE TRAVELS,

Bob Sehlinger

BOB SEHLINGER
PUBLISHER